AF574519

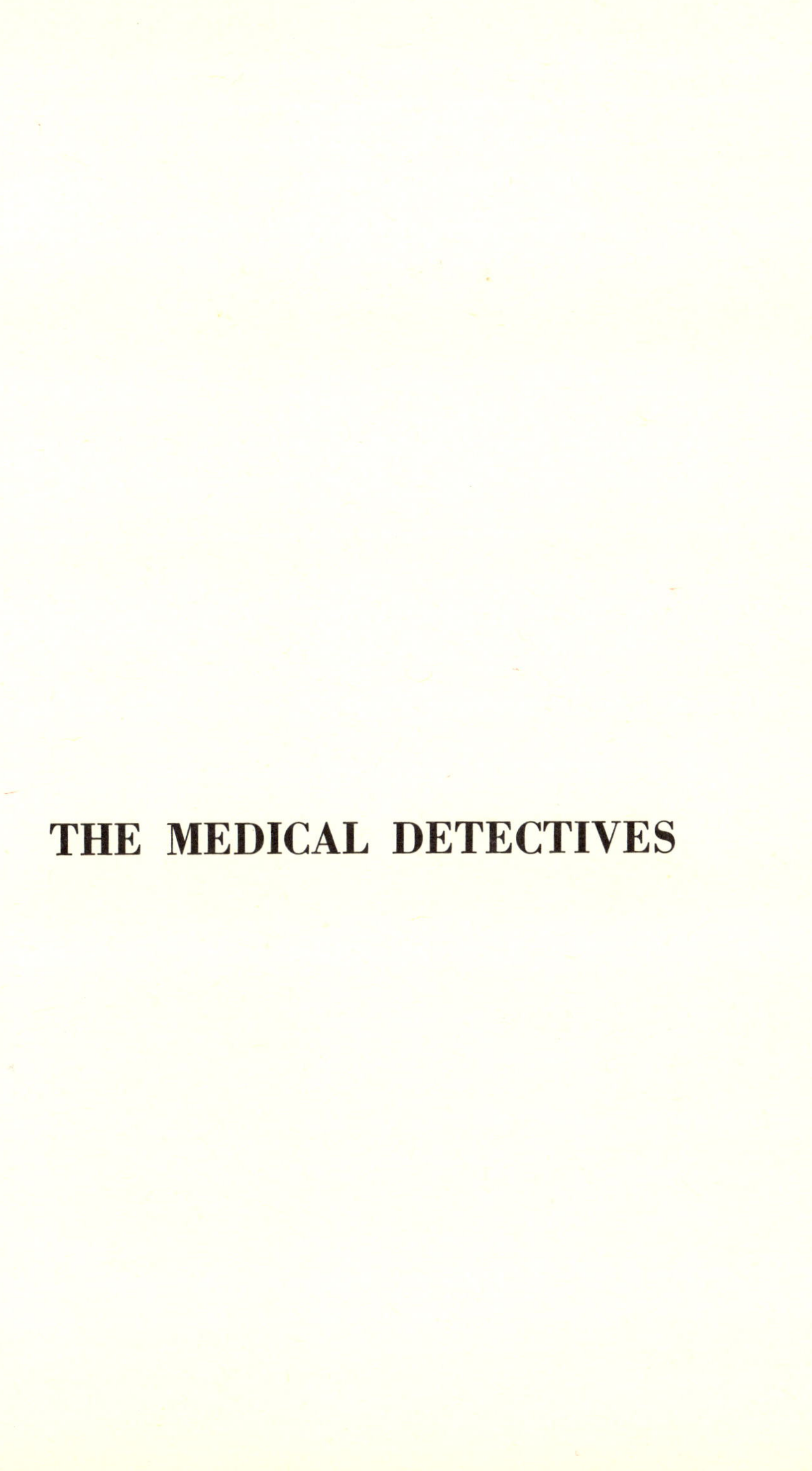

THE MEDICAL DETECTIVES

Others Books by ***Paulette Cooper***

THE SCANDAL OF SCIENTOLOGY

GROWING UP PUERTO RICAN

For Younger Readers:
HALLOWEEN

Introduction by Milton Helpern, M.D.

PAULETTE COOPER

THE MEDICAL DETECTIVES

DAVID McKAY COMPANY INC.
New York

The Medical Detectives

LIBRARY OF CONGRESS CATALOG CARD NUMBER: 73–79947

MANUFACTURED IN THE UNITED STATES OF AMERICA

ISBN: 0–679–50382–X

Dedicated to
RUCHLA AND CHAIM BUCHOLC
who died in the region of Aucshwitz. . . .

Acknowledgments

I am extremely grateful for the great deal of time given to me by those doctors who have chapters devoted to them. In addition, I particularly want to thank Dr. John Devlin, Dr. Lowell Levine, Dr. Alexander Wiener, attorney Robert Straus, and especially Dr. John Edland, who helped arrange interviews and checked this manuscript prior to publication. Listed alphabetically:

The Medical Detectives:

Dr. Lester Adelson
Chief Pathologist, Cuyahoga County
Cleveland, Ohio

Dr. Michael Baden
Deputy Chief Medical Examiner
New York City, New York

Dr. Frank Cleveland
Chief Coroner
Hamilton County, Ohio

Dr. John Devlin
Deputy Chief Medical Examiner
New York City, New York

Dr. John Edland
Chief Medical Examiner
Monroe County, New York

Dr. Harry Gordon
Professor of Pediatrics
Albert Einstein College of Medicine
Bronx, New York

Dr. Elliot Gross
Chief Medical Examiner
Hartford, Connecticut

Dr. Milton Helpern
Chief Medical Examiner
New York City, New York

Dr. M. Dorothea Kerr
Medical Investigator of the Office of the Chief Medical Examiner
New York City, New York

Dr. Judith M. Lehotay
Chief Medical Examiner
Erie County, New York

Dr. Lowell Levine
Consultant in Forensic Dentistry to the Office of the Chief Medical Examiner
New York City, New York

Dr. James Luke
Chief Medical Examiner
Washington, D. C.

Dr. Thomas Noguchi
Medical Examiner–Coroner
Los Angeles, California

Dr. Clara Raven
Interim Chief Medical Examiner
Detroit, Michigan

Dr. Abraham Rosenthal
Assistant Medical Examiner
Office of the Chief Medical Examiner
New York City, New York

Dr. Jane Simon
Assistant Medical Examiner
Office of the Chief Medical Examiner
New York City, New York

Dr. Werner Spitz
Chief Medical Examiner
Wayne County, Michigan

Charles Umberger, Ph.D.
Director of Toxicological Laboratory
Office of the Chief Medical Examiner
New York City, New York

Dr. Cyril Wecht
Chief Forensic Pathologist
Allegheny County Coroner's Office
Pittsburgh, Pennsylvania

Dr. Sidney Weinberg
Chief Medical Examiner
Suffolk County, New York

Dr. Alexander Wiener
Director, Department of Serology and Bacteriological Laboratories
Office of the Chief Medical Examiner
New York City, New York

The Legal Detectives:

Dino Fulgoni
Medical Legal Department
District Attorney's Office
Los Angeles, California

Vincent Nicholosi
Assistant District Attorney
Queens County, New York

Robert Straus
Assistant District Attorney
Brooklyn, New York

Sidney Schatkin
Attorney at Law
New York City, New York

Also:

Narciso Garganta
Medical Librarian
Milton Helpern Library of Legal Medicine
New York City, New York

Contents

Introduction

I am pleased to have been asked to write the introduction to this interesting, instructive book. A book on the work of the medical examiners provides a splendid opportunity to emphasize that all deaths that are sudden, suspicious, medically unattended, obviously violent, unusual, or that occur when a person is in legal custody, should be reported to the official medico-legal agency provided for that purpose. It is equally important that an investigation of the death be carried out automatically and not left to the option of the agency. The agency should not refuse to investigate deaths because of lack of interest or because of lack of time, and the post mortem investigation and certification of sudden, suspicious, and violent deaths should be mandatory in all jurisdictions.

At present, failure to report and investigate many of these deaths is one of the weaknesses in the system of medico-legal investigation in many places throughout the country. But that is only part of the problem. To investigate deaths effectively, agencies must have qualified, experienced medical personnel. This includes official medical investigators, forensic pathologists, and ancillary specialists, such as toxicologists—for the detection of poisons and for determining body substances—and serologists—for the examination of blood stains and body fluids such as saliva, sweat, and semen. There should be well-equipped laboratories capable of preparing tissues from an autopsy for microscopic examination, as well as facilities for bacteriological studies of deaths from infection.

It is true that not every death investigated requires all of these disciplines, and not every death requires that the post mortem examination of the body include an autopsy. Yet, it must be recognized that in addition to determining the cause and manner of death, however obvious they may appear, an autopsy is essential to establish, confirm, or provide sound answers rather than surmises to the many questions that may arise later in connection with even the most evident type of violent death.

Physicians as well as lay persons often have visited the autopsy room of the medical examiner, observed the body of a victim of a violent death by gunshot, and then asked why an autopsy was necessary when the cause of death was so apparent. When we look at a victim, apparently dead of multiple bullet wounds, we might assume without an autopsy that the wounds came from a single bullet. But on examination, if we find that they were produced by bullets of different calibres traveling in different directions, we realize that they must have been fired from different weapons, and see why an autopsy can be so vital.

An autopsy also may reveal that the stomach contents and organs of the body contain alcohol, and possibly other drugs and poisons, and while this finding may be unrelated to the cause of death, it can still provide important information which clarifies how and why the death took place. At an autopsy the presence, amount, and nature of the food found in the deceased's stomach are important and may provide a clue as to the time of death. This information may also serve as an important check on the reliability of witnesses reporting when the victim was last seen alive. In some murder cases, such findings provide the clues that point to the perpetrator.

Another determination of the autopsy, and the basis for an important, though often disregarded, principle in legal medicine and forensic pathology, is the age of the injury. A person may be seriously or even fatally injured without being immediately disabled; and death may take place after the victim has been removed from those circumstances that provide some basis for suspicion of murder. The production of symptoms from fatal wounds may be delayed, and if a careful post mortem examination is not done, or the autopsy is improperly performed, the result may be a failure to recognize the traumatic character of the death.

This ability to recognize the age of the original injury is extremely important, especially in connection with deaths caused by child abuse, or by internal or head injuries. For example, a man could meet a woman who apparently had been drinking quite a bit, take her home, and on the way witness her stumble, fall, and suddenly die. The man could be suspected of having pushed or hit her, and if the medical examiner's office reported to the police and district attorney merely that the cause of death was a traumatic subdural hemorrhage, the man could be in considerable trouble. But if it is recognized and reported that the subdural hemorrhage was at least four or five days old, and that the woman apparently had been walking around with this traumatic condition before she met the man, he obviously could be cleared.

There have been many instances in which the most obvious violent deaths, and even apparently natural ones, have been disproved by a carefully performed complete autopsy, done by a qualified, experienced, and sensitive forensic pathologist. The responsibility for detecting the cause of death is great, not only in those cases which are homicidal, but also those which are accidental, suicidal, or natural. Unfortunately, there has been too much emphasis on the work of the medical examiners in deaths which are gruesome or bizarre, and provide good copy for the mass media. Most deaths which the medical examiner clarifies by his investigation are not of this type.

For example, on a number of occasions the bleeding bodies of several victims have been found lying about rooms in which the furniture has been disarranged, so these deaths were first reported to the medical examiner's office as suspected homicides. Yet, careful autopsies have proved the cause of death to be acute carbon monoxide poisoning from an unsuspected source. In the early stages of acute carbon monoxide poisoning, when prolonged exposure to dangerous, but not heavy, concentrations of carbon monoxide in the air of the room occurs, the victim may undergo a progression of symptoms, including headache, nausea, vomiting, mental confusion, and muscular incoordination. This can cause him to stumble, fall over furniture, and knock over lamps and other objects, the broken edges of which may lacerate the skin and cause bleeding. The scene in such cases, particularly when more than one person is involved, and especially with the presence of blood, usually leads the initial observer to believe that the deaths were violent.

Strangely enough, such unlabeled cases rarely are diagnosed correctly by a physician, and not infrequently are overlooked, unsuspected, and incorrectly diagnosed even at an autopsy. Obviously it is important to recognize the nature of such deaths, for the source of the carbon monoxide may present a continuing hazard to others. The ability of the medical examiner to recognize promptly death caused by acute carbon monoxide poisoning is a good example of the way in which an effective system of medico-legal investigation can benefit the community.

This example also illustrates the fact that a medical examiner's office is as concerned with preventing deaths as with detecting homicide. It should be pointed out that the medical examiner is a guardian of the public health and well-being, responsible for detecting deaths from contagious or epidemic disease, or from poisoning in the household and in industry.

Equally important, however, is his responsibility for establishing cases in which a suspicious-looking death is not homicidal. This is important to protect the innocent person who may fall under suspicion of having committed a violent act when there was none. Clearly, the medical examiner has great responsibility for detecting the cause of death not only in cases of homicide, but also in deaths that are natural, accidental, or suicidal. It should be evident that the post mortem investigation and autopsy performed by qualified, experienced medical examiners is necessary to the proper administration of justice in any community and wherever a death becomes a subject of judicial inquiry. If anyone doubts, let him read this book.

Dr. Milton Helpern
Chief Medical Examiner
New York City, New York

PART I

WHAT MEDICAL DETECTIVES DO

1

What Done It? Dead Men Do Tell Tales

There may be no such thing as a "perfect crime" in the sense that it leaves no clues; there may be only imperfect investigators who do not know how to translate them. *Something* is almost always left at the scene. The evidence may be as small as a strand of hair, a simple spot of saliva, or maybe just a single speck of blood. The clues to be found may not even be *at* the proverbial scene of the crime but rather *in* the victim: in the chemical content of his hair and fingernails (for arsenic detection); in the blood chloride level of the chambers of his heart (to determine drowning); in the amount of carbon monoxide in his blood (for burning); etc. It is simply a matter of knowing what to look for, and understanding what is found. For it is not just a proverb but a fact that dead men do tell tales; unfortunately there is not always enough time or people to translate everything they are saying to us.

The men, and sometimes women, who find and translate these corporeal clues specialize in a field called "forensic medicine," which has been defined by its first important practitioner, an Englishman named Sir Bernard Spilsbury, as that area "where medical matters come into relation with the law." Most of us may think of these experts as "medical detectives," but their official titles are usually medical examiner, pathologist, or coroner. Some chemists, biochemists, and serologists also specialize in forensic medicine, but those who are medical examiners or pathologists must be medical doctors. In a few states coroners must be physicians, while in others the coroner can be anyone from the local mortician to the local beautician. Although the job requires an extensive knowledge of medicine and sometimes a smattering of law, it has been and unfortunately still is occasionally awarded to people who don't know a windpipe from a drainpipe.

While most states have gone beyond the old North Carolina law that stated that the only qualifications for becoming a coroner were that the person "had not denied the being of Almighty God or participated in a duel," some states still award the job solely for political reasons—although it has been aptly stated that there is no Democratic or Republican way to work on a murder or establish a suicide. The job of coroner is also given to undertakers, and at one time undertaker-coroners used to race to the scene of the crime, not to see justice carried out, but to see if *they* could carry out the body before the other undertakers got to it. Fortunately, such practices are now on the wane, and hopefully, this trend will continue as the public learns more about the role of the "medical detectives" in helping to solve crimes *and* in detection work that helps to prevent them.

Technically, the job of the medical detectives is not to solve crimes or catch criminals, but rather to provide information which ultimately is used by investigative bureaus to help *them* apprehend and punish the perpetrators. As Vincent Nicholosi, assistant district attorney of Queens County, New York, states, "The relationship between the two groups is often a symbiotic one, for the medical examiners may use the other's findings to indicate the area to look for, and the agencies utilize the medical examiner's report to show them who to look for."

Dr. Milton Helpern, chief medical examiner of the City of New York, emphasizes that "the medical detectives are not concerned with whodunit, but rather *what*-done-it," or in other words, what caused the person to die. Unfortunately, establishing this is not always simple, for, as he explains, "It's not like bookkeeping, where you add up a column of figures. Yes, you can always come up with an answer, but it may not be the right one. It's better to come up with no answer than the wrong one, for an unlabeled case is better than a mislabeled one. The important thing is to know when you don't know." Unfortunately, not all medical detectives agree. There's extremely good money to be made in giving expert court testimony, and some "pissologists," as the other pathologists call them, are all too anxious to give an opinion on the cause of death and state it as fact, when perhaps only God may know the real answer to the question.

How do the medical detectives determine the cause of death? Say a man is found dead with a rope around his neck. It would seem obvious that he had been strangled to death, or, more technically, that he had died from asphyxia or lack of oxygen. But that may not be true. Perhaps the man was poisoned to death; and since the killer knew his purchase of poison could easily be traced, he tried to disguise the cause of death by putting the rope around his victim's neck *after* he died so that no one would suspect he was poisoned. Or maybe the deceased had a heart attack as he realized that a noose was going around his neck, and the heart attack got him before his killer did.

It is therefore necessary for the medical detectives to check several things before deciding what really killed the person. The first step might be to see if the rope was pulled tight enough to kill the deceased. Next, the medical detective would check to see if the man had died from asphyxia (which *could* have been caused by the rope). This he does by looking for its classic sign: petechial hemorrhages or small, often pinpoint-sized blood spots, caused by the breaking of the capillaries from pressure and lack of oxygen. (Other signs could be cyanosis, or blue, purple, or black lips, ears, and fingertips; a protruding tongue; clenched hands, or froth emanating from the nose and mouth.)

Even if the rope was tight enough to kill and the person had petechial hemorrhages, this *still* would not prove that the rope around his neck caused asphyxiation and that asphyxiation caused his death. The medical detective still would have to establish whether the asphyxia could have arisen from other causes (such as inhaling illuminating gas, heart or lung trouble, tumors, etc.). He would have to examine all of the person's internal organs and tissues carefully to determine that none of these other problems could have been responsible for death. And, finally, he would have to establish from the appearance and size of the bruises on the neck under the rope whether the rope had been tied around the person before he died, or whether the marks on his neck could have occurred after death, perhaps from careless transportation of the body.

All this may seem like a tremendous amount of effort

just to establish a seemingly insignificant what-done-it. But determining the cause of death can sometimes cause another death—or save a life—if someone is accused or cleared of putting a fatal rope around the man's neck. Therefore the medical detectives must be certain that they are correct on the what-done-it; and that is often far more difficult to establish than in the above hypothetical example, for murderers commonly try to confuse the cause of death or lie about it outright.

For example, a medical detective once examined a woman with a knife thrust into her chest. Obviously, she had been stabbed to death. Obviously? As he examined the knife wound, he saw that it had not bled, and since dead bodies do not bleed (although they may drain, depending on the position of the person), he concluded that she must have been stabbed after she died. Guessing someone might do that in order to divert attention from the real cause of death, he examined the rest of her body carefully. He discovered that she died from the results of an illegal abortion.

As for lying about the cause of death, a man once had an affair with a young girl who lived in an adjoining state and she subsequently gave birth to his baby. The man told her he was taking the child away to his house to care for it, but instead he took it away and killed it. When he was questioned by the police as to the whereabouts of the child, he admitted to the murder, adding that he put the infant in a sack with a chloroform rag in it, drove across to his own state, and disposed of the body. He was probably conversant with criminal law, and blithely confessed, knowing that the law states that a defendant can only be tried in the state where the murder was actually committed. Who could say in which state the child had died?

And so the medical detectives were asked to help out. It appeared that the father had already given the answer to the what-done-it (chloroform), but the examiner performed a post mortem nonetheless to see if more clues could be gleaned. To their surprise, they found no trace whatsoever of chloroform in the baby's body. Had chloroform really been administered, it would probably have taken days to dissipate and so would most likely still have been found. The medical detectives therefore examined the rest of the child's body to uncover the real cause of death. The severe marks of violence on the baby's face and neck indicated that the what-done-it had been the fatal assault. When the father was again questioned and confronted with this irrefutable medical evidence, he admitted that he really had beaten the child to death. Most important, perhaps realizing that it was futile to fight further, since getting away with murder requires a knowledge of medicine as well as law, he admitted in which state he had killed his child.

In addition to accumulating evidence that may ultimately convict the guilty, the medical detective's conclusion about the what-done-it can often establish the innocence of a suspect as well. To give just one example: an automobile driver crashed head-on into another vehicle and died immediately. The accident caused serious injuries to the passengers who were with him in the car. Since the driver appeared to have been at fault in hitting the other vehicle, the passengers sued his estate. But when the medical detectives performed an autopsy on the driver, they found he had not died from the car crash at all. He had suffered a heart attack while driving, which *caused* him to crash his car. The real cause of death, therefore, stemmed from natural causes; the driver had not been at fault, and the surviving passengers could not collect from him.

The basic tool of the medical detectives which ultimately can convict the guilty and vindicate the innocent is the autopsy, and if more autopsies were done, more killers would be convicted—or more innocent people acquitted. Unfortunately, there is neither enough time nor enough specially trained medical personnel to perform an autopsy everywhere in the country on every case that might require one, although it should be pointed out that not every death warrants it. In fact, autopsying every person who dies would be as foolish as arresting every person seen on the street at the scene of a crime.

As a result, the medical detectives must learn to recognize suspicious signs, or disparities between a person's condition and the official reports of his death. Sometimes the medical detectives literally cannot put their fingers on exactly what is wrong; but a good one instinctively knows when something is the matter. As Milton Helpern states, "If I have to stop and ask myself *whether* I should perform an autopsy on someone, then I *have* to do one. If I didn't suspect that something was wrong, I would never have asked myself that question in the first place."

The cynical may say that to perform an autopsy is useless, for it is too late to be of value once the person is dead. Is he really helped if his killer is caught and convicted? Or if his family is relieved when they learn that his death was not a suicide? It is, of course, true that an autopsy does nothing to help bring back the deceased, but the finding of the medical detectives can prevent death and injustice to the living. If a murderer escapes, he may feel confident enough to murder again. If a person commits suicide but is believed to have been murdered, innocent people may be sent to jail—and have been executed—for the "crime." If an accidental death is mistaken for suicide, someone in the family who feels responsible may take his own life as a result of the guilt. And as the final chapter will show, society in general, and not just those related to the deceased, often can be helped by the discoveries made in autopsies.

An autopsy can be valuable even when there is no question about the what-done-it, as is shown in this final case. It had its beginnings when an attractive woman entered a doctor's office, and, amidst sobs, told him that she had become pregnant despite all precautions. The doctor listening to this story sat back in his chair. He had heard this one before. How often had these girls come to him, asking for an abortion? This was not the problem. The difficulty was not that she was in need of an abortion, but that she had just had one. She told the doctor that after the operation, which she said had been performed in another part of the city, she was walking home and had suddenly become extremely ill. She stopped—collapsed, in fact—at the first doctor's office she found. His luck it had to be his. He said later that he had asked the girl for the name of the doctor who had performed the illegal operation but she refused to tell him. He had to stop questioning her when she began hemorrhaging profusely. A few minutes later she was dead.

The medical detective who came to this doctor's office found the woman lying dead on the couch with no evidence of any recent operations having been performed in the office. He realized that this doctor's story might well be true, but he also knew that it would be a good way for the doctor to explain away a patient who had died on his hands, as he was performing the abortion. What if there were no first doctor and this one was literally trying to get away with murder? Although he knew the what-done-it, he decided to perform an autopsy to see if he could find some clues.

He found one. Chloroform had been used as the anaesthetic, and the girl still had 156 milligrams of chloroform per 1,000 grams of brain. The medical detective compared the choloroform rate in other anaesthesia cases and found that in a person anaesthetized for minor operations, the chloroform content is between 120 and 182 milligrams in 1,000 grams of brain.

Now, the doctor had said that the woman claimed to have walked to his office from another part of town. But if a person is anaesthetized by 120 to 182 milligrams of chloroform, and the victim's brain contained 156 milligrams, she obviously was too heavily drugged to have been able to walk from the one office to a second. It was apparent that there had been no first doctor; that *this* one must have administered the chloroform in his office for the abortion. As a result of the autopsy findings, the doctor did several years in prison, probably regretting most of that time that he had not stated that she was carried into his office, and most likely also regretting that they had not taught him more about forensic medicine in medical school.

A large part of the medical detectives' work described in this book (most has never been revealed before) was done in the field of criminology. While medical detection in the areas of rare diseases, epidemiology, or occupational poisoning has become known through the commendable writing of Berton Rouché, most Americans, including the criminals, know very little about medical detection in criminology. It is not only a fascinating subject but an important one. In almost all of the cases presented in this book, the criminal thought he could get away with his crime because he was unaware that there was a medical way to detect his deed. Perhaps as the work in this field becomes better known, it will cause some people to think twice before trying to commit a so-called perfect crime.

2

How Was It Done? The Brides in the Bath

The following case took place in England at the turn of the century and is still the classic case in forensic medicine today—and one of the most fascinating. Although in America it is usually the criminal who is showered with publicity, in England it is often the medical detective as well. This case brought into prominence Sir Bernard Spilsbury, the greatest pathologist in English history, who captured the public's interest and made it aware of how exciting was the work of the medical detectives. Today, there is still a great fascination among the English in medical-legal matters, and the average layman there knows more about forensic medicine than some lesser experts here. The interest all started in 1901, after a young woman died in her bathtub. . . .

George Joseph Smith was a man who only took one bath in seven years. It wasn't that he didn't like baths; the truth was that he was obsessed with them. But he only seemed anxious to have his *wives* take a bath, especially right after he married them—provided that their inheritance and insurance would ultimately accrue to him. The reason Smith didn't bathe himself was that he believed that bathtubs were dangerous places, and he ominously commented on more than one occasion that people had been known to die in them. He certainly was in a position to know. Three of his wives died in their bathtubs.

The police were first apprised of the suspicious situation when they received a short news clipping about a woman named Margaret Elizabeth Lofty, who just one day before this article was written had married a man named John Lloyd. The two had been married in the English town of Bath. The couple had traveled all morning by train to reach their honeymoon site, and at the end of the day, when Margaret complained to her husband of a headache, her bridegroom dutifully took her to see a doctor, who diagnosed the flu. Her husband's concern for her health was probably a relief to her, as was the unexpected marriage, even though she had to admit that her new husband was patently not the romantic type. His idea of a marriage proposal had been to ask to look at her bankbook.

Still, Margaret Lofty, a masculine-looking brunette, was thirty-eight years old and had never been married before. When she met Lloyd, she had just recovered from an unhappy love affair, portentously enough with a man who turned out to have been secretly married all the time. She never lived long enough to find out that Lloyd, whom she had known only briefly before the marriage, was also secretly married—indeed to several wives at once. Perhaps it was merciful for her that she never had a chance to learn the truth about his background, for her flu, combined with the hot bath, caused her to faint in her tub that night and drown. At least that is what the doctor wrote on her death certificate.

It appeared that Lloyd had nothing to do with her unfortunate accident, for the landlady heard splashing from the bathroom above, and a few minutes later she heard someone, whom she knew could only be John Lloyd, playing the organ for ten minutes. He chose a funereal composition. Yet a few minutes later, Lloyd rang the front doorbell and told the landlady that he had been out for a while. He then inquired as to the whereabouts of his new wife. If he was grief-stricken on learning that his bride of one day was dead in her bathtub, he showed no signs of it, and later ordered the cheapest possible coffin.

Surely he could have afforded a little better. The will that Margaret Lofty had drawn up only three hours before she died brought him $2,000. He made money from more than just her insurance, for he had spent his first and only afternoon of their married life with her, unromantically enough, at the bank, where she had withdrawn her entire savings account and transferred it into his name. Shortly after her death he profited even more by selling all of his bride's clothes and possessions, not even sparing the linens she had left at the laundry—these he sold before they were returned, and never paid the laundry bill.

The police investigation which led to most of these discoveries (the news clipping had been very brief) also uncovered the fact that Lloyd had evinced an obvious and unnatural interest in the bathtub of the rooming house before signing the rental agreement. Indeed, he may have been the only bridegroom in history to spend a greater proportion of time studying the qualities and dimensions of the bathtub than the bridal bed. Other people noticed this strange concern as well, for another boarding house on the street had turned him away because of this unaccountable obsession. After all, not every potential boarder rings the bell and asks the landlady if she has a bathtub before asking if she has a room, then examines the tub for a quarter of an hour, comments that a person "could lie down in it," and proceeds to test this to see if it's true—while fully dressed.

Still, while Lloyd's behavior was eccentric, it did not prove that he was responsible for his wife's "accident" in the bathtub. The whole situation would probably never have been investigated in the first place, except that the police received another news clipping together with the one about the death of Margaret Lofty.

The second article had appeared one year earlier in a different paper. It told the story of a similarly hapless bride named Alice Burnham. Alice, an attractive, buxom, twenty-five-year-old girl, had been married for only six weeks to a man she had barely known, named George Smith, and she too had suddenly accidentally died during her nocturnal ablutions. Like poor Margaret, she too had suffered from a headache the day before her death and like Margaret's husband, hers solicitously had taken her to a doctor, who later said that the heat of the water must have affected her heart, causing her either to faint or have a fatal fit in the tub.

Here, too, Smith had made some not-so-discreet inquiries about the bathtub before he had rented the place, and he had rejected an earlier house on learning it contained no tub. Upon discovering that this wife had died in the bathtub—and again he seemed to be out of the house when she died, for he rang the front bell and said so—he removed his coat and rolled up his sleeves before lifting his beloved from the bathtub. Like Lloyd, he showed no sorrow, bought a cheap coffin, and defended this thrift by the matter-of-fact statement that "when they are dead they are done with." Afterward, he tried to beat paying the rent and then vanished.

Smith had proposed to this wife in his own unique manner, bringing Alice Burnham his bankbooks and papers, and then insisting on seeing hers in exchange. It was unfortunate for Alice that he didn't instantly leave her when he saw that this potential bride had no money. Instead, he waxed eloquent on the benefits of love, marriage, and insurance policies, and convinced her to take out a $1,000 life insurance policy, and name him as the sole beneficiary.

Smith, like Lloyd, was not the kind to leave any stones unturned, especially if there might be money for him under them. When he found out from Alice on that romantic night that she had loaned her father about $250, Lloyd waited until after he married her and then immediately ordered the father to turn over the money to him. With interest.

From the moment Alice's father met his future son-in-law, he took an intense dislike to him, based initially on his appearance, for there was something sinister in Smith's eyes that instilled physical fear in the prospective father-in-law. Mr. Burnham saw that his fears had some basis in fact when Smith wrote him a series of semiliterate letters ordering him to pay up the money, containing veiled threats about Burnham's safety, and opened threats of litigation, if he didn't fork over fast. When his daughter died and Smith lied to him about the time of the autopsy to keep him away, Burnham became convinced that his daughter's death was no accident. It was Mr. Burnham who by chance came upon the news clipping of the other bride who had died in the same manner as his daughter, and he lost no time in sending both clippings to the police.

Yet despite the two clippings which were so sinister in their similarities, and despite all that the police had discovered in their own investigations, they still did not know the whereabouts of Lloyd or Smith. Furthermore, they could not be certain whether the two men were the same, although the description of each—medium build, around forty years of age, with piercing eyes—tallied. They realized that there was one sure way to reach Lloyd (or Smith) fast, and that was to mention his favorite word: money. So they got in touch with Margaret Lofty's insurance company, which had been suspicious enough of the circumstances surrounding her death to withhold their payment on her insurance policy. The police told the company to try to reach Lloyd and tell him that they had changed their minds and all was well—he could collect his money. Then they waited.

When a medium-sized man in his forties, with piercing eyes, arrived at the insurance office, a detective casually asked if he was named John Lloyd. This he affirmed. The detective then asked Lloyd if he was also known as George Smith, which he vigorously denied. Without any show of concern, the detective nonchalantly explained that he had asked this question because they were checking up on a slight technical difficulty since Lloyd had used two different names on his two marriage licenses. When Lloyd heard he was only being questioned for something minor, and not murder, he breathed a sigh of relief and admitted he was both Lloyd and Smith. The detective also breathed a sigh of relief, and hauled Lloyd-Smith away to question him about the death of his two brides. The detective knew it would be hard to prove that Smith had murdered them, but he knew enough about forensic medicine to realize that if he could not prove murder, perhaps Sir Bernard Spilsbury could.

George Joseph Smith (which turned out to be his real name) had a criminal record starting at the age of nine, and a long history of swindling women under the aliases of Lloyd, Williams, Baker, James, and, inappropriately enough, Love. Murdering for money was a late development in his criminal career. Before, he had learned how to get money from women without any murderous machinations. He sent his first wife out to work, and then convinced her to steal from her employers. Obviously, she had trouble getting references afterward, but to solve that problem, Smith did his only work during that period: he posed as her former employer and provided her with phony credentials. When she got caught with stolen goods on her, Smith disappeared quickly, literally leaving her holding the bag. But she was one of his few wives to get her revenge, for she told the police how Smith had cheated for her, a statement which resulted in his incarceration.

When Smith got out of jail, he realized it was time to change his approach. Instead of having women steal for him, he stole from *them.* Some of these women he married, while others he just dated, but his method was the same regardless. First, he would try to acquire her possessions and money with persuasion. Failing that, he would take her out to a park or museum (which of course was free), leave her there "for a minute," under some pretext or other, and then race back to her home and steal all of her possessions.

There was one wife, however, whom Smith treated differently, and whom he seemed genuinely to care for, since he lived with her intermittently for seven years, returning to her whenever he was idle between marriages and murders. But he was no more generous with her than with his other women: once, when he ran off and left her for a five-month period, he sent her five dollars to keep her going.

Why the women Smith married would trust such a monster, or even like him, is a mystery, but women found him so appealing that even after his deeds were known, they flocked to his court trial to get a glimpse of him and hopefully even touch him. As is often true in these cases, he was neither distinctive-looking nor attractive. His one outstanding feature was his eyes, which seemed to cause women to melt and men to recoil. Smith was practically illiterate, although no one could ever say he was stupid. He thought Germany was spelled with a "J," but as shall be seen later, he invented an entirely new method of murder, almost undetectable, to anyone but Spilsbury. It is true that his wives' deaths aroused suspicions, but that would never have happened if he had waited longer after marrying to execute the murders, for newspapers will always pick up a story about a bride who did not live through her honeymoon.

Smith was also a mean and miserly man and the only money he didn't begrudge spending on his wives was for insurance policies, doctors, and lawyers. He beat those of his wives who lived long enough, and would humiliate them in various ways. He locked one of them in the closet once for several hours, and deliberately married a woman he planned to kill in a bath in a town with the same name—Bath. Even after he had murdered his wives he treated them cruelly, for instead of covering them modestly, he seemed to derive a perverse pleasure in flaunting the naked bodies of his brides to the landladies, neighbors, and police. The only wife he treated with any "kindness" was the one he often lived with, and probably the best thing he ever did for her was to advise her not to take baths. That Smith himself avoided baths probably is not surprising, considering the sinister use for which he thought bathtubs were intended.

Still, perhaps there was one good thing that could be said about George Joseph Smith. Unlike murderers who get colder and more callous with each killing (as is often the pattern), Smith was probably cruelest to his first victim, and later showed a bit of tenderness to his wives before murdering them. But the police only found this out after he was arrested for the other two murders, for it was only then that they learned that a few years earlier there had been *another* man, named Henry Williams, whose wife had *also* died in her bath, and in this case Smith (alias Williams) had reached his nadir.

That story started when a man who called himself Henry Williams briefly courted a thirty-three-year-old woman with false teeth named Beatrice Mundy, who was not particularly ugly, but certainly not attractive either. There was no doubt that it had been love at first sight from the moment Williams found out that Bessie had money. A few hours after the marriage ceremony, he demanded that she give it to him, but she honestly explained that the $5,000 inheritance she had told him about was untouchable. She could only collect the interest from it, which came to about twenty dollars a month. Still, the marriage was not a total loss for Williams, for about $300 of this interest had been resting idly in the bank. So he seized the accumulated interest, plus all of her clothes and possessions, and left her with what she was born with.

Williams then blamed his abandonment on her, and wrote her a letter claiming he had left because she had given him venereal disease, or the "bad malady," as he put it to her in his letter. But he was kind (if unsophisticated) enough to suggest that she might have contracted it from unclean personal habits rather than from an unclean lover. (Then too, he simply may have been trying to set things up so he'd have an easy time getting her into a bathtub later.) His letter also carefully instructed her to spend none of the interest that would continue to accumulate from her inheritance, and to save it all for the day when he would return to her. In the meantime, unbeknownst to her, he went back to live with his favorite wife.

Williams was probably planning to return when Bessie's interest would begin to interest him, but apparently by accident, Williams bumped into Bessie two years later at a resort town. While a less lonely or foolish woman would have recoiled from a man who had treated her in such an egregious manner (or would have called the police), Bessie forgave him and took him back after less than two hours of lies and persuasion on his part. Shortly thereafter, Williams went to see a lawyer and asked him if he would become the sole heir to Bessie's money if she should suddenly die. The lawyer's affirmation was the wife's death knell. Six days later, Williams got Bessie to draw up a will which made him the sole beneficiary to her $5,000.

By then everything was set, but the crucial prop in his play was still lacking: the bathtub. He had had less foresight in these early days, since the place they were living in had no tub. So he sent *her* out to buy the bathtub he planned to kill her in and gave her strict instructions to bargain down the price and purchase it only on credit. He never did pay for the tub, for he returned it to the store four days later, after his nefarious use for it was over.

Williams again appeared to have been out of the house when the landlady downstairs heard some splashing, a gasp, and then saw water trickling from the ceiling as if the bathtub had overflowed. Again, Williams found a doctor who wrote off the death as accidental, for he had previously taken his wife to a physician lest her death later seem suspicious. Williams had told that doctor that his wife suffered from epilepsy, and he also convinced Bessie that she had seizures without knowing it. Her only complaint to the doctor was that she suffered from a headache.

After her death Williams did evince enormous grief and wept at her funeral. But the effect of his act was lost when he suddenly turned off the water like the little Dutch boy who put his finger in the dike, and cheerfully asked, "Was it not jolly good that I got her to make out a will?" Williams did not have the decency to use part of her $5,000 to at least get Bessie a cheap coffin. He had her buried in a common grave, which cost him about a dollar. He did spend some fifteen dollars for the funeral, but he got much more in return by selling Bessie's piano and furniture to the undertaker.

So at last the police had the entire picture. Smith had married three women in four years, all of whom had died shortly after the wedding. Each death had occurred in the bathtub. The doctors—who were almost as foolish as the wives in this case—had all seen the wives earlier and then attributed their deaths to accident. Lloyd-Smith-

Williams never seemed to be present at the time of death, but made a point of coming in later from outside. Did the brides in the bath die naturally? By accident? By suicide?

Or was it murder? There was certainly sufficient circumstantial evidence to support that conclusion, but unless Sir Bernard Spilsbury could prove that it was homicide—which meant that he had to show *how* their deaths could have occurred—George Joseph Smith was free to walk out of prison and find himself another bride.

One of the most important things a medical detective must establish after the what-done-it is *how* a person died, that is, whether the death was a result of natural, accidental, suicidal, or homicidal cause.

While this NASH classification, as it is called, is helpful, it has inadvertently characterized suicide as a crime. The classification originally arose because of the necessity to assign blame to every death: either God or man was responsible. All deaths caused by man had to be punished, and while this certainly should be true for homicide, it has unfortunately been extended to include suicide. For centuries, suicide has been punished by mutilation of the body after death, sanctions on the place and manner of burial, and forfeiture of his property. Old English law stated in addition that a suicide had to be buried on the side of the highway with a stake driven through the heart, perhaps in hopes of keeping the ghost from haunting the living. Today several states in America still have laws on their books which make suicide or its attempt a crime, and, even in the so-called more enlightened states, the suicide and his family are sometimes stigmatized.

Still, without this NASH classification, justice—and the insurance companies—could never prevail. Even when the medical detective easily can establish the what-done-it (as in the above case, which appeared to have been drowning), if he comes to the wrong conclusion on the how-was-it-done, or the manner of death, injustice can ensue. For example, if he mistakenly classifies a homicidal death as one of the other three categories, a murderer may go free. If a natural, accidental, or suicidal death is erroneously believed to be homicidal, then time and money can be wasted searching for a nonexistent killer. If an accidental death is ascribed to something else, the deceased's family may not collect their due on a double indemnity accident insurance policy clause; and if a death is inaccurately attributed to suicide, they may receive no money at all. Besides which, the pain and shock that a person undergoes if accused of murder (when there is none), or that a family feels if told that a member committed suicide (when he did not), or that a man feels if he believes he was responsible for an accidental death (when he was not), is inestimable, and often irreparable.

Sometimes, establishing the how-was-it-done follows naturally from the what-done-it. For example, strangulation with a ligature is usually homicidal. But in other instances it may take more work for the medical detectives to figure out the how-was-it-done than to establish the what-done-it. Still, the how is often just as important as the what, for it may determine if one should look for a who-done-it. If a death is due to natural or accidental causes, usually no blame is ascribed to anyone. But if death is suicidal or homicidal, someone is always responsible (in suicide it is the person himself).

As a result, if the what-done-it proves to be a blow on the head from a rock, and the rock turns out to be a meteorite, the how-was-it-done is probably accidental, and no further investigation would be made. But if a person was hit on the head by an ordinary rock in a lonely park at night, the blow probably did not come from the sky.

When the how-was-it-done is believed to be homicidal, an attempt is obviously made to find the killer. Naturally, many murderers, instead of hiding the cause of death, try to mask the circumstances of the killing so the medical detective cannot tell how it was done. This is easiest to do with asphyxial deaths. If a parent kills his baby by compressing its chest with his own body until the infant suffocates, no physical signs may reveal how asphyxiation occurred. Or, if the victim was lying face down on a soft mattress and his assailant pressed him down with a pillow and smothered him to death, no physical signs may disclose the asphyxiating instrument. When murderers do this, while the medical detective usually knows that death came from asphyxiation, he cannot tell if the asphyxiation was homicidal, suicidal, accidental, or even natural, and the killer may get away. After all, no one may even realize that there *was* a killer.

Murderers often try to make homicide look like suicide, although they sometimes give themselves away by their lack of medical knowledge. One man hit his victim on the head and then placed him beneath a low bridge to make it appear as if the man had jumped to his death. He was caught when the medical detective saw that the deceased had been hit in *two* places on the head, and concluded that no one commits suicide by jumping off a bridge twice.

Although the medical detectives must know how to detect unsuspected homicide, it is just as important for them to be able to determine when no murder has taken place despite suspicious events. They do this by carefully searching for corporeal clues that show that what at first glance may appear to be homicide, at second scrutiny turns out to be far less sinister. Just as murder can often look like suicide, accident, or even a natural death, the latter three categories of death can likewise look like murder.

Natural deaths are occasionally mistaken for murder; suicide can easily be confused with homicide. Almost every method a person could use to put an end to his own life can be used by someone else to end it for him. The only exception is manual strangulation, for a person cannot deliberately asphyxiate himself with his bare hands (although he can with a ligature). He falls unconscious before dying, which causes his hands to relax, restoring the circulation of blood to the brain. But a person could die from a heart attack by trying.

Accidental deaths also sometimes may look like murder, as happened once when a woman on a ship went overboard. Although there was no question that the what-done-it was drowning, the severe bruises on her body made it appear as if she had also been beaten. Suspicion immediately fell upon her male companion during the voyage, who was suspected of having beaten her for some reason and then pushed her to her death. The medical detective, however, realized that it was probably an accident, for he noted that her bruises lay solely on one side of her body, and he knew that no one could beat up a person so selectively. Yet such marks were perfectly consistent with a fall from a height into water.

When some medical detectives examine a body in which something does not look right, they immediately suspect homicide, while others first look for signs of less sinister nature. Dr. Milton Helpern, who probably comes closest to being the Spilsbury of America, has spent as much time affirming natural and accidental deaths that initially look suspicious as he has in detecting homicides that no one else suspected. (He has absolved the innocent in many cases, including the man under suspicion in the case of the woman who fell overboard.)

On the other hand, Dr. Thomas Noguchi, the boyish-looking coroner-medical examiner for Los Angeles, immediately starts with the supposition that "everything is murder unless proven otherwise." This approach has validity too, for as he explains, "Once you make the mistake of considering a murder to be an accident, you burn your bridges and can't go back because the chain of evidence is broken." He cites as an example the case of what looked like a simple automobile accident in which a car burned up. While the driver escaped unharmed, the woman who was in the car with him was killed. Since it was presumed to be an accident, the woman was cremated without an autopsy and the car was destroyed. Only later was it learned that the driver had a quarter-of-a-million-dollar accident insurance policy. Moreover, his house had burned down three times and three times he had collected on the insurance. But by then the car was gone, the woman was dead, and so little concrete evidence remained that a case against the man resulted in two hung juries and he never could be convicted.

Like Dr. Noguchi, Sir Bernard Spilsbury was the suspicious type. He took one look at the exhumed bodies of Smith's three no-longer-blushing brides, perused the report on the doctors' conclusions about the how-was-it-done, tossed it away, and literally screamed "murder!" His first task was to make certain that the what-done-it definitely had been drowning, and that Smith had not first killed his wives by other means and placed them in their bathtubs later.

To see if someone has drowned, the medical detectives usually compare the blood chloride levels of their left and right heart chambers. If they are the same, the most likely conclusion is that the person was killed before he ever entered the water; if different, he probably drowned. The reason for this is that the water and fluids which enter the lungs are carried around to the left chamber of the heart. If the person dies, the circulation suddenly stops, and only one chamber is filled with water. Other indications of drowning are aspirate material in the heart, stomach, and microscopic flora in the lungs, etc.

Although Spilsbury confirmed that the what-done-it was indeed drowning, he still was faced with the more difficult problem of how. There is no physiological way of determining whether someone held a person down under water unless physical signs of a struggle are found on the body. Usually the only clue that the drowning was accidental and not homicidal comes from the circumstances. If a person drowns under very strange conditions—for example, drunks and epileptics have been known to drown in small puddles—it was probably an accident, since no killer (or potential suicide) would take a chance on using so little water.

Spilsbury's first hypothesis, that Smith had drugged his wives in order to slip them under the water, was disproved when the toxicological report showed no drugs in their bodies. Spilsbury knew that Smith's next most likely method was physically to force the women under the water, but it is hard for a man to pin down a grown and struggling woman without leaving some bruises on her body. Spilsbury had found only one small mark on the left elbow of one of the wives, along with two small bruises beneath the surface of her skin. These apparently had been caused so soon before her death that they had not had time even to appear on the surface of her body.

Yet Spilsbury had, as evidence of violence, the testimony that two of the landladies had heard splashing; in one case the water from the tub had overflowed; and several hairs from one of the wives had been found against the back of the bathtub. It was obvious that Smith had somehow got these women under the water so fast that they never had time to scream or struggle, and it was unlikely that he could have done this just by holding them down.

Spilsbury also wondered about the fact that Bessie Mundy was clutching a piece of soap when she was found. Now, Smith had set up the situation so that it would look as if his wife either had fainted or had a fit in the tub which caused her to slide under water while bathing. Spilsbury knew that if the first was true, namely that Bessie had fainted, she would then have released the soap as she became unconscious and she would have died empty-handed. The fact that the soap was still in her hand indicated that she had had a cadaveric spasm, or muscular reaction, at the moment of death, and clutching the soap was her final act. Therefore, she must have died without ever losing consciousness. This suggested that she had not fainted.

As for the other theory, that she had had an epileptic fit in the bathtub, Spilsbury did not think it was likely. For one thing, he knew that many epileptics utter a warning scream before their attack, and the landlady had not heard Bessie shout out. In addition, Spilsbury was told that she never had had epilepsy before her marriage to Smith, and he knew that the possibility of someone's first getting it as they approached the age of thirty-five (especially a woman) was unlikely. Most important, he realized that none of the three phases of epilepsy would have caused her to sink down in the water in the position in which she was found. On the contrary, the first tonic phase causes the body to stiffen, which would have thrust her up, and she would then have been found leaning forward in the bath, not backward, as they found her.

The position in which all three brides were found was suspicious for other reasons as well. For one thing, if the women had bathed in a manner consistent with the way they were found, they would have gotten their hair totally wet while bathing. Most women try not to wet their hair while in the tub, unless they are washing it, and none of these women were. Spilsbury sensed that the position in which the women were found was crucial, and in order to make further analysis, he asked the police to trace and send to his office the tub in which Bessie had been drowned. He immediately realized that it would have been very difficult for her accidentally to have slipped down and drowned in it, because she was seven inches bigger than the tub. In fact, she had been found dead with her feet draped over the end. And that was another thing that bothered Spilsbury: he knew that people who are too big to fit into their bathtubs usually do not stick their feet *out* of the tub but rather curl themselves up or flex their knees in order to make themselves fit. Spilsbury kept thinking about that one: Why were her feet over the tub in such an unnatural position?

And then all at once it hit him. Her feet were over the tub because Smith had *put* them there. Although his ultimate goal was indeed to get their heads in the water, he probably did it by pulling their feet out first. Smith must have either yanked his wives' ankles so fast that their heads went under before they realized what was happening and could try to stop him, or else he may have put one arm underneath their knees and the other under their heads as if he were preparing to lift them out of the water. If he then had jerked their knees up fast, this would have caused their heads to slip under the water immediately. Either method was consistent with their general posture, and could account for Bessie's feet being found over the bottom of the tub as they were. Spilsbury knew that sudden entrance of water into the nose and throat would cause immediate shock and would most likely leave no real physical injuries, since death would come too fast for the victim to struggle.

In order to test his theory of how it was done, Spilsbury hired a female swimmer who was the same size as Bessie Mundy. He had her get into the same tub, and when her ankle was pulled, she went down without a struggle. But Spilsbury's satisfaction over discovering how Smith's wives had died was cut short when Spilsbury saw that the model was also drowning in the water. The method was so successful that she had become immediately unconscious from the sudden entry of water into her nose and throat. Fortunately, since she had been prepared in advance for what was going to happen, and she was a strong swimmer, she survived. Still, it took thirty minutes before she was revived, although it took the jury only twenty-two minutes to condemn Smith to a much less imaginative death than the one he had invented—hanging by a rope.

PART II

CLUES FROM THE CORPSE

3

What Blood Reveals: The Crazy Carpenter and the Sheppard Case

It was late in the afternoon of July 1, 1901, when two little German boys suddenly disappeared from the Baltic island called Rugen on which they lived. The boys were Herman Stubbe, who was eight years old, and his six-year-old brother Peter. They were both typical Nordic children—blond and blue-eyed—who spent most of their days in school, and then often went to play with their schoolmates for a few hours before going home to dinner.

Their father had no objections to their playing, but he often admonished them against using the woods as a playground—not because he thought that any people lurked there, but because he knew that dangerous animals did. But like all young boys, Herman and Peter were often wont to disobey. Not that there was anything special to do in the forbidden woods, but doing anything that was forbidden at that age is always special.

Their father first sensed that something might be wrong when his two sons failed to return home in time for dinner. Although they were usually punctual, at first he was not alarmed unduly by their tardiness. He remembered what it was like to be young, and he simply assumed that the two boys were most likely playing in the woods despite his warnings, and had either lost track of the time, or, more ominously, the way. But when his sons still had not returned home late that evening, the father got the sole policeman on the island and some neighbors to form a search party to go out in the woods and look for them. The group gave up early in the morning, discouraged and defeated, seeing no signs whatsoever of the children.

After a few hours of sporadic sleep, the search party continued its work the next morning. The search was suddenly over when the two boys were found—dead. Their bodies were uncovered in some shrubs, and the rock with blood on it found nearby indicated how they most likely had met their fate. Death always comes as a shock, especially when it happens to young children, but the condition in which these two little boys was found made the incident even more sickening. Their heads had been brutally bashed in and were severed from their bodies. In addition to the decapitation, the killer had torn off their arms and legs, slashed their bodies open, and, like Jack the Ripper, crudely vivisected them. The missing organs—minus the heart of the older boy, which was never found—were strewn over a wide area in the woods and were found a while later. And as a final indignity to an already heinous crime, the little boys had been the victims of a brutal sexual assault.

The residents of this tiny town talked of nothing else, but despite all of their concern and gossip, it was hard to elicit much concrete information on the activities of the children prior to their disappearance. While people wanted to do everything possible to help, few people in the town knew either the children or their father, since the three were living in Rugen only for the summer while the father was employed at a hotel in this resort town.

Fortunately, there was a fruit peddler in Rugen who had come to know the little boys, and he remembered seeing them late on the afternoon of their disappearance. He told the magistrate that he had noticed them talking to an itinerant carpenter from a nearby village, a man named Ludwig Tessnow, the proverbial village idiot and a source of amusement with his strange speech, lopsided gait, and odd mannerisms. Later that day, a man who worked on the roads volunteered that he too remembered seeing Tessnow that night, but not with the children. Tessnow was alone, and the workman had noticed even in the dark that his light dress suit was splattered with strange brown spots.

The town magistrate lost no time in finding Tessnow and bringing him in for questioning, but that was about all he could do. Tessnow denied knowing the two boys, talking to them that night, and most certainly killing them. The magistrate made the carpenter produce his two sets of clothes, and he noticed that while neither set was clean, the dress clothes looked as if they had been washed recently. The act had not been entirely successful, for there were still some barely visible dried spots on the shirt, hat, jacket, trousers, and vest lining. But the carpenter was adamant that they were wood, not blood stains, and plausibly explained that when he had to dye light wood, it was impossible for him not to get a few stains on his clothes.

The magistrate was suspicious, as he knew that laborers do not usually work in their dress clothes, but his investigation nonetheless had reached an impasse. There was no way to prove that these faint stains really were blood and not dye, for in 1901 little was known about medical detection and blood evidence. There were only a few medical detectives at that time and they were mostly working in large cities, not in places like Rugen. Furthermore, to those who did not know better, their work seemed to have little practical value, since they were only at the stage of testing their theories in laboratories.

One of the sciences they were just beginning to explore was called serology, and forensic serologists were just starting to develop ways to distinguish blood stains from less sinister ones like dye and paint. It was not an easy job, and even today, despite all that has been learned, mistakes are made in macroscopic (as well as microscopic) examination. Many stains which appear to the naked eye to be blood ultimately prove totally innocuous. Blood is only a bright red hue when fresh, or when seen in movies or on television in order to make it easy to discern on a color set. In real life, if a bright red stain is found some time after the death, the one thing that is probably certain is that it is not blood, which can be dark red, brown, gray, yellow-green, or even colorless.

Usually, however, there is not much blood around to see—regardless of its color. While it may be a bloody nuisance to them, most murderers know that it is well worth the extra time to ensure that no trace is left at the scene, on themselves, or on their weapons. But even if they cannot see any blood around, those more sharp-eyed and sharp-witted have found it—seeped through the cracks of a wooden floor, slipped into the space between the knife blade and handle, or encrusted in the tiny incised name of the knife's manufacturer, among other places. One murderer, who washed all of his garments so thoroughly that not one visible drop of blood was left, was caught by the blood that had seeped into the nail holes of his shoes' rubber heels. Another man, who had an ax to grind with a friend, used that weapon to kill him, but since he knew that such a murder would leave a lot of blood on his clothes, he didn't wear any. Obviously the examination of his clothing revealed nothing, but he was eventually convicted because blood was found caked under his toenails.

Even if the blood lost at the scene literally cannot be spotted, the tests that have been developed to establish whether it was once present are so powerful that, as Lady Macbeth found out, no amount of washing can totally eradicate the evidence. A murderer once transported a corpse in the trunk of a car, then scoured the trunk with detergents, ran water through it for twenty-four hours with a hose, and then painted the incriminating area with red lead. It *still* gave a positive sign for blood when tested.

Even when blood undeniably is present, and the suspect is confronted with this irrefutable fact, he usually will try blithely to attribute its source to something innocent. It is common in rural areas for people who are accused of murder and found with suspicious stains to insist that it came from slaughtering an animal. (As shall be seen later, this is easy to prove or discount.) Some more sophisticated murderers are wise enough not to resort to the old animal alibi, but hang themselves by falsely attributing any blood on them or their clothes as emanating from a nose bleed, or as a result of having intercourse with a menstruating woman. (On the other hand, if a man denies raping a woman but has her menstrual blood on him, he insists with equinoctial regularity that the blood came from a nosebleed, cut finger, etc.) But medical detectives today know how to determine the precise source of blood from a body.

Blood from a nosebleed is admixed with nasal mucus; menstrual blood has a high acid content from vaginal mucus and contains vaginal epithelium cells and numerous microorganisms. Moreover, the location of the blood on the assailant can give a clue as to its source. Dr. Cyril Polson, a British medical detective, reported that one murderer insisted that the blood found on him was a result of making love with a menstruating woman, but the man couldn't for the life of him explain what position he had used for intercourse that would account for the blood found in his armpit!

Much can be learned about a crime not only by analyzing the location of the blood from the victim, but also by studying the location of the blood at the scene. To cite just a couple of rules, a lot of blood around indicates that the victim probably survived for a while after the attack, for dead bodies do not bleed. Bleeding stops when the heart is no longer pumping blood through the body. If the blood is spread over a very large area, then the deceased most likely was mobile after the injury. (This may not seem important, but it can indicate the difference between a suicide and a homocide, since suicides are usually stationary while waiting to die, there being no reason for them to struggle or move around.)

Sometimes the location of the blood is the only remaining evidence that can show what really happened. A man once admitted to killing his wife by striking her on the head with an iron, but he insisted he did it in self-defense while she was threatening him with a butcher knife. When he hit her, the blood from her head had spurted on the wall, so the distance of the blood from the floor was measured. Its point of origin was eighteen inches off the floor, and her head could be that low only if she was already down when he struck her—hardly an act of self-defense.

One other type of test which the medical detectives apply to blood today—and which often proves crucial—is typing it into the four main groups (A-B-AB-O) to see whose blood it is. The results are usually used to acquit a suspect rather than convict him, because millions of people belong to the same group. Thus, even if the blood on a suspect is the same as that of his alleged victim, it could have come from someone else. So if a suspected murderer has type A blood and his alleged victim has type B, if type B is found on the suspect, this may put one more nail in his coffin but it does not close the lid. If the blood on him turns out to be type O, however, it could not have belonged to the deceased. Incidentally, a person who has on him the blood type of the person he is accused of killing cannot change his blood grouping to try to get around this. If he totally transfused his blood with someone else's, his body would manufacture a replacement supply with its same old grouping.)

Even when there is no blood left to be found and typed, serology is now so advanced that it is possible to type substitutes. Approximately 80 percent of the population are "secretors," and the grouping substances of their blood exist in their perspiration, saliva, semen, vaginal secretions, urine, bone marrow, mother's milk, and hair. This grouping is invariably the same as the blood group. A man with type B blood, therefore, cannot have type O semen. The agglutins and agglutinogens are most concentrated (and therefore the easiest to type) in saliva; a cigarette smoked dry, saliva on gags, and bite marks, all have revealed the blood type of the person. Once, by grouping the saliva *on a postage stamp,* a suspect who belonged to a different blood group was eliminated.

Often, substitute secretions have been used in murder cases. For example, blood stains were once found on a suspect's jacket which were not of his group, but the victim's blood type could not be determined because she had been embalmed, i.e., her blood was removed. The police reported that they had noticed that she had sewn small perspiration shields into the underarms of all of her clothes, so the medical detectives set about extracting the perspiration from them. From this, they easily were able to establish her blood type—which was the same as that on the suspect's jacket.

This grouping is often used in sex crimes, to see if the semen in or on a woman (and sometimes on a man from the reflux of semen) is of the same group as that of the alleged rapist. By grouping the stains on clothes, it was once established that a woman was telling the truth when she said that three men had intercourse with her (although that did not prove her accusation of rape). And since the three semenal groups of the men had become mixed with her own vaginal secretions, the medical detectives could determine in what order the three had coitus with her.

At the turn of the century, though, none of this was known, and even the basic step of distinguishing animal from human blood or even blood from other stains had not yet been reached. Jurgen Thorwald, who first uncovered this case, said it was not the first time that someone suspected of murder and found with suspicious stains on his garments had insisted that they were wood stains and not blood. Three years before the Stubbe boys were murdered, on September 8, 1898, a similar murder took place in another town in Germany called Lechtingen, not far from the boys' town of Rugen. On that day, two little

German girls, Hannelore Heideman and Else Hangemeier, had, like the Stubbe boys, failed to return home at noon for their meal. The girls' parents went to the school to see what had delayed their children, and learned that neither girl had been in school at all that day.

They, too, made a thorough search of the woods, thinking that the children might have stopped to play on the way to school and then lost their way. These two little girls were found dead—one underneath some bushes, the other hidden under a pile of twigs. This murder also had been gruesome, with the children's organs removed and scattered around the woods. Suspicion had fallen likewise on a carpenter, who naturally insisted that the stains on him came from dyeing wood. Since there was no way to prove otherwise, the carpenter was released and the case remained unsolved.

The magistrate in Rugen was totally frustrated by his lack of progress in the Tessnow case, but he would not give up. Knowing what had happened to the two little German girls a few years earlier, he wrote to the magistrate of the girls' town to see if there had been any new developments in that case which might help him with his. He learned that the investigation into their deaths also had reached an impasse, and that the magistrate of that town had long since given up. But he learned a startling piece of information which strengthened his conviction to solve this crime: the carpenter who had been questioned and released in connection with the death of the two little girls was named Ludwig Tessnow.

Now, the magistrate was convinced that Tessnow had committed the murders, not just two, but four. Since he had something tangible (if circumstantial) upon which to base his suspicions, he initiated a full-scale investigation into the murder of the Stubbe boys. One fact initially seemed to have no connection with the rest of the case: on June 11, a couple of weeks prior to the murder of the two little boys, half a dozen sheep had been killed in that same southeastern area of Rugen where the boys had been found. When the magistrate learned that the sheep had not been killed by an animal but by a person who had then slit them open, disemboweled them, and scattered their organs around the field, he knew he had hit upon something important.

The magistrate immediately questioned the man whose sheep had been killed, and the farmer said he had seen the slaughterer fleeing in the dark after his act. He was sure he would recognize him if he ever saw him again. When the magistrate brought Tessnow over to him, the farmer studied his strange walk, the disjointed movement of his arms, and his unique profile, and concluded that Tessnow was definitely the man he had seen fleeing after killing and mutilating his sheep.

But even with this information, there still was little the magistrate could do. Before forensic serology had developed, a man could kill two girls, two boys, and various animals; if he was not caught in the act, he could get away with it if he insisted that it was not their blood which had been found on him. There was just no way to prove otherwise. But this magistrate refused to quit. He had kept up with new developments in criminology and he remembered reading about a strange new science in which it was said to be possible to look at tiny spots through some peculiar machine and determine if what was being looked at was blood. Furthermore, it was said that it could be determined whether the blood came from a person or from an animal—and sometimes even what species of animal. So late in July, the magistrate sent Tessnow's two sets of clothes and the bloody stone to one of "those big city places" and asked them to ascertain what kind of stains were on the garments. Were they wood or blood? And if the latter, did they come from a person? From an animal? Or both?

Tessnow's clothes, which contained nearly a hundred stains, were examined by a military doctor named Paul Uhlenhuth, only thirty years old at the time. Yet he had devised a method which could identify and distinguish blood stains from people and animals. His discovery had been published in February of that year, just in time to help convict the children's murderer.

Uhlenhuth examined the stains on the clothes, treated them with his complicated method, and reported to the disappointed magistrate that the stains on the carpenter's work clothes really *were* wood stains and not blood stains, just as the carpenter had insisted. But the stains on Tessnow's dress suit were another matter. While some of those stains had been too small to work on (a problem forensic serologists still sometimes face), others were capable of analysis. Uhlenhuth discovered that sheep's blood existed in nine places on the dress clothes—and human blood in twenty-two.

Before any more German children could be killed to satiate his perverse desires, Tessnow the carpenter was duly convicted and executed.

Since 1901, when the two little Stubbe boys were found, serology has advanced far beyond the point of establishing whether or not a stain is blood. Unfortunately, people's attitudes have not always progressed at the same rate as science. It was not so very long ago that a white woman in the South was found murdered, and shortly thereafter, a black man was seen with blood on the sleeve of his jacket. Despite the paucity of evidence, the townspeople screamed that obviously he was responsible, and refused to believe or even listen to his explanation that the blood had been the result of a recent hunting expedition. It was only after he was lynched that anybody bothered to ask the medical detectives to check whether it was human or animal blood. It was animal blood. The woman's true murderer later turned out to be her husband—who no doubt had led the lynching mob.

But injustices have occurred not only because of prejudice. Within the last fifty years serology has become a complicated science which has given rise to many self-proclaimed experts in the field, some of whom know little. For example, it is axiomatic that if a person is running while bleeding, the blood usually will appear in the form of an exclamation mark, with the period at the end of the path of blood. Dino Fulgoni of the medical Legal department of the District Attorney's Office in Los Angeles, who is extremely knowledgeable about forensic medicine, was trying to question (or discredit) a very weak serological expert for the defense. "Do you know what happens to blood when someone's running?" Fulgoni asked the so-called expert. "Sure," he replied, "it falls down."

Thus, it is not surprising that justice sometimes miscarries due to misinterpretation and lack of knowledge on the part of the "experts." In one such case the "victim" was Dr. Sam Sheppard, a thirty-year-old osteopath who lived in Bay Village, Ohio, a small suburb near Cleveland.

Despite some difficulties, Sam Sheppard, married for nine years to his high school sweetheart, Marilyn, seemed happy with her. He admitted he had been involved in an affair, but he was no longer seeing the girl. Marilyn, on the other hand, had found intercourse painful after the birth of her son seven years earlier, and her sex drive had decreased. However, she was now pregnant again, the baby due in five months, and she and Sam were discussing returning to a double bed as they had in the early days of their marriage. They also enjoyed financial comfort. Sheppard earned more than $30,000 a year, owned his own two-story waterfront home in Bay Village, a Jaguar, a Lincoln Continental, plus a half-share in a boat, and he seemed well on his way to fulfilling his high school prophesy as the Man Most Likely to Succeed.

Everything changed some time during the morning of July 4, 1954. The night before, Sam and Marilyn had watched television with close friends, during which time Marilyn ensconced herself cozily on Sam's lap throughout the show. This scene was interrupted when Sam received an emergency call, and he went out to work for several hours in a futile try to save one young patient's life. When he came home, he fell asleep on the downstairs couch, totally exhausted. He claimed that he was awakened while still on his makeshift bed by noises from the upstairs bedroom, and hearing his wife scream, moan, and call him for help, he dashed up the stairs. He thought she was having problems with her pregnancy, similar to those she had suffered from while she was carrying their son, but as he entered the darkened bedroom, he saw someone standing by his wife's bed. Leaping on the person, he was hit from behind on the back of his neck, apparently by another person in the room. That blow caused him to pass out, and when he regained consciousness, the assailants were gone.

So was his wife. He immediately took her pulse, and saw that she was dead—totally battered and bloodied from what later was determined to be thirty-five vicious blows, primarily on her face and head. He had no time to grieve for his wife, or for the child he would never have, for after he had checked on his son in the next room (who was unharmed), he heard a noise downstairs. He dashed down, and then chased a man out the back door and down to the beach in back of his house. He claimed that he fought with him briefly before he was knocked unconscious for the second time that morning, and that he did not revive until water from the incoming tide swept up over him.

At a quarter to six in the morning, he called his closest friend, who was also the part-time mayor of the town, and told him: "Come quick. I think they've killed Marilyn." The mayor and his wife arrived a few minutes later and found the place looking as if it had been burglarized. Sam was seated in a chair with wet slacks, holding his neck with his hand, and seemingly in great pain. The mayor made a few calls. A policeman was the next to arrive, followed by Sam's brother Richard, also an osteopath. According to the mayor, Richard asked Sam whether he had anything to do with the murder, although Richard later denied that he had ever asked or even thought such a thing. When Sam's other brother, Stephen (yet another osteopath), arrived a few minutes later, he also inadvertently harmed Sam's cause. He examined his brother, found that he had serious neck injuries and suggested that he immediately be hospitalized. Later it was said that his family had "spirited him away" lest the police question him—although they questioned him bluntly and relentlessly in the hospital anyway. Sam was accused of either faking his injuries or inflicting them upon himself.

Primarily for these reasons, Sheppard was accused of committing the murder. The *Cleveland Press* and the Cuyahoga County coroner were particularly certain of his guilt, although neither should have been allowed to play the role of prosecutor. The *Cleveland Press* may have subscribed to the adage that crime doesn't pay, but it does sell newspapers. They carried lead articles and editorials proclaiming that Sheppard was being given preferential treatment because of his money and his family's connections, and headlined their opinions with such subtleties as "Getting Away with Murder," and "Why Isn't Sam Sheppard in Jail?" Even when things died down, and the prosecutors and public lost interest in the case, the *Cleveland Press* was there, fanning the fire with inflammatory stories of Sheppard and his "guilt."

The other "prosecutor" in this case was Dr. Samuel R. Gerber, the coroner of Cuyahoga County. He sometimes seemed as anxious to stay on top of the news as on top of his job, as when, for example, he posed for the newspapers holding up Marilyn's bloody pillow and pajamas. Actually, Gerber appeared to be eminently qualified to testify in forensic matters, since he had degrees in both law and medicine. But this was a complicated case requiring a great deal of expertise in serology. Marilyn Sheppard's bloodstains, which drenched the room, might have told the entire story of the crime, but only to an expert in this area. Blood interpretation has become so complicated since the turn of the century that unless one is an expert, it is like looking at the blots in a Rorschach card: a person can see whatever he wants in it, and there's room to project one's own personality and prejudices into the blood blots as well.

There were two trials in the Sheppard case. Although there was no question in the trial as to the what-done-it (blows) or even the how-was-it-done (murder), the crucial question during the first trial was with what, for no weapon was ever found. The prosecution contended that during the time that Sam claimed he was unconscious, he was disposing of the murder weapon. Actually, the weapon used was not important in this case, but it was made so by the prosecution, and the wrong answer led to the wrong who-done-it. The type of weapon should have been determined by examining Marilyn's bruises, but Gerber "analyzed" the shape of the copious bloodstains on her pillowcase, and decided for some reason that the murderer had put the weapon down on the pillow for a short time and her blood had poured over it. There was no doubt in Gerber's mind that the pattern that was left showed that the weapon had been a "surgical instrument," which clearly left its "blood signature" on the pillow. Obviously, this was very damaging, actually devastating, for Sheppard would be assumed to own a surgical instrument while any other intruder would not.

Gerber went even farther. He said that the surgical instrument was two-bladed, about three inches long, with teeth on the end of each blade. F. Lee Bailey commented years later that "there hasn't been a surgical instrument like . . . [that] since the days of Hippocrates." And in the second trial in the 1960s, Bailey got Gerber to admit that he had no idea of what kind of surgical instrument he had once so knowledgeably described, and that in fact he never actually had seen any instrument like it. That was the end of the surgical instrument hypothesis, just as surely as that preposterous theory had nearly been the end of Sheppard.

What harmed his case in the first trial almost as much as the surgical instrument was the prosecution's final witness, a twenty-four-year-old laboratory technician, who admitted that she had been Sam's former mistress. Introducing her into the case was an overt attempt to provide a motive to the murder, but its real purpose was more subtle. While adultery was against the law, in the eyes of the jury it was even worse. Her revelations about their relationship changed the case from a court trial into a witch trial, as the prosecution tried to lead the jurors to conclude that someone who commits adultery would have no qualms about committing murder. Unfortunately, even in the twentieth century, there are those—including jurors—who believe this.

Sam was found guilty of murder. Later, more blood evidence was accrued and analyzed by a renowned expert and the Sheppard case was reinterpreted. Unfortunately that did not occur until after the trial in 1955, when Dr. Paul Leland Kirk, a Ph.D. biochemist and one of the foremost criminologists in America, stepped into the case. While Gerber had devoted scant attention to the blood in the bedroom (he was only supposedly in that room for three minutes), Kirk wrote in his report that "the most significant evidence . . . was the blood distribution in the murder room."

In order to understand the case better, Kirk built a model of the bedroom with moveable walls and pieces of paper to represent blood. The first thing he found was that there was a large spot of human blood located in the bedroom which was neither Sheppard's type A, nor Marilyn's type O, implying that a third person probably was there and injured during the struggle. (This supported Sam's claim that there had been someone else in the room early that morning who hit him.) Kirk was able to establish where the killer had been standing: behind that area was the only place on the wall with no blood on it, which meant that a body had intercepted the splashes.

Kirk figured out which blood spots on the wall had spurted from Marilyn's head as she was struck, and which spots came from the backswing of the killer's weapon as he repeatedly lifted his hand to strike again. This information, in conjunction with the position in which Marilyn was lying and the place where the killer was standing, showed that the murderer was left-handed. *But Sheppard was right-handed.*

Kirk studied more than just the blood in the room. He knew that another important piece of blood evidence lay in Sheppard's clothes, and he paid careful attention to Sheppard's belt and shoes because blood can never be completely removed from leather. With one exception, there was absolutely no blood on Sheppard's clothing, and while the prosecution had hinted in the first trial that Sheppard had washed his clothes in the lake that night, if Sheppard had put them under Niagara Falls for two days he could not have removed totally the amount of blood that would have splattered on him from the thirty-five vicious blows to his wife. The single exception, the one blood stain on the clothing, was a small smudge on his left trouser leg, and this supported Sheppard's story that he had leaned over Marilyn's bloody body to take her pulse that morning.

As for the murder weapon, Kirk studied the photographs of her bruises and concluded that the most likely villain was a flared-end flashlight. Gerber may have concluded that a surgical instrument was the weapon because the pillow had a strange, almost even pattern of blood, which is atypical of the usual amorphous bloodstains. But Kirk felt that the pattern came either from Marilyn doubling the pillow to ward off the blows, or from the killer doubling it to place it over her head to stifle her screams.

Kirk even found a possible motive for the murder.

Marilyn had been found with her legs outspread, her breasts bared, her pajama top pulled up, and the bottoms down. Kirk believed that it was probably a sex attack, and that this was the motive and not the cover-up, i.e., someone did not kill her for one reason and then try to make it look like a sex attack later. He based this on the fact that the largest amount of blood had accumulated at the bottom of her legs, showing that her pajama bottoms had been pulled down before she was beaten. Otherwise the blood would have been primarily on the pajamas. A sex attack probably also ruled out Sheppard, since not many husbands rape their wives, or at least have to beat them to death in order to get them to copulate.

From that evidence, and more, it appeared that Sam Sheppard really was innocent. But it was eleven years before he was permitted to have the second trial which proved it. By then, it was an empty victory. He had already lost his wife and future child and never had the satisfaction of knowing who really had done it. He spent a decade in prison for a crime he probably did not commit. His mother, who was broken by the two-month-long trial which stamped her son as a murderer, committed suicide seventeen days after Sheppard was convicted. Eleven days later his father, who had lost one of his sons, his daughter-in-law, his future grandchild, and then his wife, died of a bleeding gastric ulcer. Sam's in-laws never spoke to him again after their daughter's death, and Marilyn's father committed suicide while Sheppard was still in jail. Sheppard spent his time in jail knowing that his son was spending his formative years without parents, and was being continually ridiculed and maligned by his peers for being the son of a killer. Although Sam Sheppard had been very close to his two osteopath brothers before Marilyn's death, the pressures caused the close-knit family to disband and not speak to each other when he got out of jail.

Things began to change and the world started to look good to him again when he fell in love and became engaged to a beautiful blonde German divorcée with whom he had been corresponding while in prison. But within a few days the papers reported that his fiancée's half-sister (who had been dead for twenty years) had been married to Goebbels, with Hitler the best man at the wedding. So once again Sheppard became the object of public scorn and hatred—although that did not stop him from marrying her.

When he returned to his former profession of osteopathy, a patient's family sued him for malpractice and the hospital in which he had performed surgery for negligence, charging that the hospital should not have allowed him to perform an operation when he had not practiced in ten years. The newspapers picked it up, and soon the families of two other patients sued him as well. Not surprisingly, the hospital's insurance company threatened to cancel its policy unless the most (in)famous doctor was dismissed, and Sam resigned. Naturally patients were scarce when Sheppard tried to go into his own practice.

Exactly one day after he left the hospital, his pen-pal wife sued for divorce. They divorced, he became a wrestler, and then he married his wrestling manager's daughter, who was less than half his age. From the time he got out of jail he drank heavily, perhaps to wash down the pills he was also taking, and on April 6, 1970, he died, at the age of forty-six. Some say he died of cancer; others that it was a combination of liquor and pills; the official coroner's report attributed it to "liver failure." Misinterpretation of blood evidence had convicted him; reinterpretation had acquitted him; either way, Sam Sheppard lost.

4

What Time Will Tell: The Beach House Murder

The police received a call one day stating that an unidentified boy of about twenty had been found in an isolated beach cabin, which was known to be the site of frequent drunken brawls. When they got there, they saw that the cabin had been totally wrecked, and an enormous amount of blood had been spilled in the room. They had no clues as to who might have killed him, until one of the neighbors reported that a particular man had been seen leaving the cabin about thirty-six hours before this boy's body was discovered. They found and arrested him, but things got more complicated when the police received a second tip from someone else who had seen a couple leaving the cabin some twelve hours before the body was found. The medical detective checked the degree of rigor mortis and reported to the police that the boy had been dead for at least six hours when found. Was the first man or the couple that came later responsible for the murder? And how could the medical detectives decide?

Medical detectives have many ways of determining the date of death in terms of days, weeks, or even months. Although some of the clues they utilize are physical, some of the best turn out to be extracorporeal. Dated mail may be lying in the mailbox; the degree of coagulation of milk in the refrigerator can be measured; the condition of food or its remains on a table can be analyzed. Newspapers often provide an indication of the date, and this is true not only for those papers which have accumulated outside of the door, but also those used to wrap up a murdered body. It is amazing how many people trying to dispose of the victim in an otherwise meticulously planned "perfect crime" erred by wrapping the body in that day's newspaper, virtually trumpeting the date of the murder. (A few of these losers have given away the location of the murder as well, for murderers who have traveled for miles to dispose of a body in order to avoid detection will use their local newspaper as wrapping paper.)

When a body dumped in the woods or fields is not found for a while, the season of the death can be deduced by examining the vegetation underneath the deceased. While everything around the person may continue to grow normally, the blossoms, leaves, and vegetation on which he was placed are crushed and killed.

When medical detectives have to establish the time of death in terms of hours, however, the clues generally are neither as clear nor as plentiful. Sometimes, in violent deaths such as a car crash, fall from a height, or fatal assault, the deceased's watch may stop or be shattered, which is a lucky break for the medical detectives. Usually the clues are subtler. If a person dies during the night the medical detectives may check his bladder. Since most people urinate before they go to sleep, an empty bladder suggests death shortly after the person retired. If a man dies in the daytime, the medical detectives may check the condition of his beard. The average man's beard grows regularly at the rate of about 0.15 mm. a day. If the person shaves solely in the morning, a heavy growth suggests that death occurred late in the day, although this is valid only for the first twenty-four hours after death; after that the skin shrinks, making a person's beard and hair look longer than they did in life. This is the basis for the popular superstition that hair, beards, and nails grow after death.

Stomach contents can often reveal when a person died. If the time the deceased ate his last meal is known, the amount of food left in his stomach and its degree of digestion can show how long he lived after eating. An unidentified, apparently transient woman once was found beaten to death in a small town. In her stomach the medical detective found spaghetti, ravioli, and olives, which he realized were the vestiges of an Italian meal eaten before her death. Fortunately it was a small town. There were only two Italian restaurants, and one of the waitresses remembered seeing a woman who fit the description of the unidentified dead woman. Although she knew nothing about the woman herself, she did know the name of the local man she was with in the restaurant. When they found and questioned him, he did not deny that he had dinner with the woman, but he insisted that he had left her—alive—about an hour after the meal. The medical detective, however, knew that the food had not yet left the woman's stomach to enter the small intestines, and that digestion had barely started. Although gastric emptying is dependent on fat content of a meal, alcohol intake, and age of the individual, he could tell that she had died *less* than an hour after completing her meal. When the man was presented with this evidence, he admitted that he had killed her.

The best-known way of determining time of death is by the degree of advancement of rigor mortis. That usually begins three to six hours after death, is complete in about eight, and passes away in thirty to forty hours. (Actually, different doctors give different times for its onset, duration, and cessation. As one of them said, "Just about anything you say about rigor mortis is correct.") It first manifests itself in the eyelids, then the jaw muscles, neck, face, chest, arms, trunk and legs, and it disappears first in the muscles in which it started. Unfortunately, there is enough variation in time between the different steps that it can usually only provide a range, and movies or books in which a doctor peers at a person and pontificates that "rigor mortis shows that he died thirty-two and one-half minutes ago" are as ridiculous as the fact that half of these so-called doctors do not even touch the body before arriving at their so-called conclusion.

Another commonly used indicator for time of death is the person's body temperature. Once a person dies and his body stops producing heat, he cools slowly to the temperature of his surroundings within a certain period of time. Unfortunately, there is no easy equation to determine rate of cooling. Body temperature is affected by the deceased's obesity (fat people cool slower), his clothing (naked people cool faster), his age (adults cool slower than children), his health, his position, and the weather outside. It is also sometimes affected by another variable—the murderer.

In one case in England, the coroner discovered that the body temperature of the deceased was close to zero degrees Fahrenheit. That would not have presented a problem necessarily, except that it happened to be colder than the coldest day in England that year. It was suspected that the murderer had put the person in a refrigerator in order to obfuscate the time of death, an apparently successful ruse, since the case remains unsolved.

Despite its limitations, though, body temperature is often used to fix the hour of death, and under some circumstances—such as when two or more people die at different times—it may be one of the best tests. As an example: a boy once told the police that he had come home, had a fight with his parents, and then killed them in succession. He later denied his own testimony, and said that his father had killed his mother, and that when on returning home several hours after the murder he had discovered this, he lost control and killed his father. Which story was true?

Both parents were found dead in the same bedroom. If the boy had killed them one right after another, it would seem their body temperatures would have been approximately the same. But there was a great disparity in degrees, and the mother's was the lower one, indicating that she had been dead longer than the father. Thus the son's second statement, that he had killed his father later, seemed to be supported. But then the medical detective looked around the room and noticed that the mother had been lying on the bed next to an open window, while her husband's body lay across the room. This completely changed the picture. Since her body had been exposed to the cold air, she would automatically cool faster than her husband. Thus, they probably both were killed at the same time. The boy was convicted.

Although the importance of time of death has been highlighted and limelighted mainly in cases of murder, it has also proved critical in less sensational modes of death, especially where insurance is involved. Someone who wants to commit suicide and has an insurance policy that only pays out for suicide one or two years after acquiring the policy, may wait for the day after the policy expires before ending his own life—and the insurance companies want the medical detectives to be sure that the insured did not miscalculate the date.

Time of death can likewise be important in accidents, as, for example, when a husband and wife are both accidentally killed in the same car crash and each has a family from an earlier marriage. Whether the husband or the wife dies first may determine which family inherits the money. Even in natural death, the time it happens can make a difference, as when, for example, someone goes to sleep before midnight, dies sometime during the night, and has an insurance policy which expires at precisely midnight. This is not a hypothetical situation, for such cases actually have happened.

The time of death of several people, and not just one or two, can sometimes solve a crime, or, as in the following case, help to prevent future ones. Dr. James Luke, the chief medical examiner of Washington, D.C., noticed that he was getting no drug death victims for a few weeks, then suddenly four or five in one week, and then the cycle would repeat itself. He drew a chart, establishing exactly when the drugs were hitting the streets of Washington, D.C., and with this information, the police were able to catch a ring of drug pushers.

Finally, in addition to determining exactly when a person or several people were killed, the medical detectives must sometimes determine when the fatal wounds were inflicted, or when the attack was initiated. In most instances, this requires analysis of the blood or bruises, although if rape is also part of the crime, or is the crime itself, there is an additional indicator—the amount of living spermatazoa in or around the victim. For example, a European policeman once had to transport a seventeen-year-old offender (probably a prostitute) from one town to another by train. Midway to their destination, however, instead of changing trains as he was supposed to do, the policeman took the girl to a movie, rented two rooms at a local hotel for the night, and waited for the next day's train.

The next day the girl refused to continue on with him, and claimed that he had raped her the previous evening. He denied having intercourse with her, but sperm and menstrual and vaginal secretions were found on the sheet—incriminating evidence, especially since she was having her period. Most incriminating, however, was the state of the sperm that was found. It was known that this woman had had intercourse about twenty hours prior to the time that the policeman took her to the hotel room. It therefore remained to determine whether this semen was the reflux of the earlier act, or semen that had been forced on her by the policeman.

A considerable amount of living spermatazoa was found on the sheets. Not many would have been alive more than twenty hours after her earlier sex act. In addition, a menstrual period accelerates the elimination of sperm from the vagina. The other possibility, that the semen could have come from someone who had occupied the same room before them, was negated when the hotel keeper proved that the room had not been occupied for two weeks, and that the bed linens had been washed during that time. The policeman was found guilty.

As to whether the first man or the second couple killed the boy in the cabin, remember that the boy had been dead for at least six hours. At first glance, the couple who had been seen leaving the cabin about twelve hours before the murder would seem to be the killers. But this case shows why the medical detectives must establish when the fatal wounds were first inflicted, as well as when the person died. From the appearance of this boy's injuries, and the large amount of blood he lost (remember that dead bodies do not bleed), taken in conjunction with the age of the blood (which can be determined at the scene by drawing a pencil through the blood to see if it leaves a mark or is covered up by the liquid), the medical detectives determined that the fatal wounds were inflicted at least a day before he died from them. Therefore, the second couple must have arrived after he was stabbed. It was the first man who killed the boy.

5

Corporeal Clues: The Cincinnati Strangler

When a middle-aged mother of three children was found raped and strangled in Cincinnati, Ohio, on December 3, 1965, few people realized that the murder was the first of a series of such rape-stranglings paralleled in current history only by those of the Boston Strangler. But on the day that Mrs. Emogene Harrington was found dead with a thin, yellow plastic clothesline wound tightly around her neck, the only indication that this was part of a pattern that would be repeated six times lay in the assault six weeks earlier and four blocks away on a sixty-five-year-old woman who survived a rape, beating, and attempted strangulation with a clothesline. Even so, what happened to Mrs. Harrington that day probably would have received scant attention in the press, except that her husband, Dr. R. Paul Harrington, was a well-known man, the head of the University of Cincinnati's aerospace engineering department and employed previously with NATO and NASA research projects.

The newspapers, therefore, splashed the story of this

short, friendly, dark-haired fifty-six-year-old woman, who had been found at one-thirty in the afternoon in the basement bathroom of her apartment house. The janitor found her, which was ironic, for she apparently met her death while looking for him, since he usually carried her heavy groceries into the apartment for her. It appeared that she had entered the basement to look for him that day, for her groceries were still locked in her car when she was found. (Robbery might have been the motive since the change from her purse was gone.)

The janitor called the police, and the police immediately called in Frank Cleveland, the tall, lean, crew-cut Hamilton County coroner, who, like all coroners in Ohio, is a physician. This was the first of the strangling victims he was to work on. Ultimately he and the police would gather a lot of evidence—he in the area of how the murders were done, they in the area of who might have done them.

On this first murder, he established that Mrs. Harrington had been dead for less than an hour when she was found, that the cause of her death was strangulation by that clothesline, and that semen and internal injuries indicated that she had been raped.

He tried to check the assailant's blood type from the semen, but failed because the semen was mixed with her blood. Still, he could tell by the bruises that she first had been beaten, then dragged inside the bathroom, where she was raped and strangled. He could tell that she was raped before death because the wound reaction on the body differed from the type of reaction that appears after death.

Unfortunately, he could tell little about the assailant from the strangulation because he had used a ligature. If a strangler uses his hands, the direction of the attack can sometimes be determined by the type of bruises on the neck: an attack from the front will leave thumb marks on the front of the neck; an attack from the rear will probably leave no thumb marks on the tough skin at the nape of the neck, but will leave severe fingermarks on the front of the neck. The wounds on the neck of a strangled person may also show the spread of the assailant's hands (an indication of his size). In theory the fingernail marks provide a clue (well-groomed nails, which leave even marks, suggest higher socioeconomic status than rough nails). It is rare, however, to find a perfect crescent from a fingernail, because the victim usually moves in his struggle.

Dr. Cleveland found two clues which helped link this murder to the earlier assault. The first was the rope used to strangle Mrs. Harrington. It had loops at each end which the killer had made for his hands. The attacker of the first woman, striking likewise in a dimly lit basement, had made the same loops in the clothesline.

The second clue was found during the autopsy. Admixed with Mrs. Harrington's own dark hair was a foreign hair which seemed to belong to her assailant. This was important. While no one can be hanged by a hair, since individual hairs differ so much from each other that no one can ever determine beyond a doubt that one hair definitely belongs to one particular person. On the other hand, some people have literally been saved by a hair, because it can be conclusively demonstrated that a particular hair definitely *could not* belong to a certain person. Hairs can also tell something about the person within a broad range—such as sex, age, and race—and thus can be useful to the medical detectives.

Dr. Cleveland sent the hair to the FBI laboratory, which, utilizing a technique called neutron activation, revealed that it was the pubic hair of a black man. The hair and the rope suggested that Mrs. Harrington's attacker was probably the same black man whom the first victim had described; a man thirty-five to forty years old, about five feet, four inches tall, with a medium build.

Other than that, nothing was known about the murderer. The police tried to trace the clothesline and found it was common cord that could have been bought at any one of the five large local supermarkets. After a while Cincinnati forgot the stranglings, for no further clues turned up in the next few months, and neither did other victims.

It was almost four months later that the next middle-aged woman in Cincinnati was found raped and murdered. She was Lois Dant, a fifty-eight-year-old mother of a nun. Mrs. Dant had always been a cautious woman, and after the Harrington murder was even more careful than usual to keep all of the many locks on her doors secured. It did her no good. One morning each week her husband left her alone, and one day when he returned he failed to find her in the basement laundry room of the apartment where she said she would be. He rang his back bell, and when he received no answer came around and let himself in the front door. He found his wife dead in the living room.

Again Dr. Cleveland was called in, and this time he found the victim on the floor with her black and white polka-dot dress pulled up, her underclothes ripped off and placed under her body, and her shoes strewn nearby. There was blood on her face from the blows of an undetermined heavy object, and she had been dragged and then strangled with a stocking. During his on-the-scene investigation, Dr. Cleveland found one stocking hanging in the bathroom which matched this one, so he told the police that there was no need to trace the murder weapon. In fact, the only difference between this crime and the other was that the killer had not come with a prepared weapon but improvised one at the scene.

Dr. Cleveland gave as the time of death a period between nine-thirty and ten-thirty. Mrs. Dant's cousin later reported to the police that she had been talking with Lois Dant on the telephone at about ten o'clock that morning when Mrs. Dant suddenly interrupted the conversation and said that someone was knocking at her front door. She told her cousin to hold on while she checked it out, and then she returned saying that someone had asked her how to find the apartment manager.

Although the newspapers had printed that the first victim—the one who survived—had been approached by the assailant under the guise of asking for directions, Mrs. Dant was not suspicious: her first floor apartment was frequently mistaken for the manager's and she commented on the fact to her cousin. She continued her conversation for a few more minutes and then said that someone was again knocking on her door, prophetically adding that perhaps that same man had returned. It was just about then that the wife of a retired detective living upstairs said she had heard a loud noise of either surprise or fear—and then the slam of a door.

Again, Dr. Cleveland ascertained that the victim had been raped, and from that fact he was able also to extract another clue. He typed the semen and learned that the killer had type O blood. Later, he found black pubic hairs which matched those found on Mrs. Harrington's body. By now there was obviously a pattern, and also obviously a crazed killer loose in Cincinnati.

He struck again two months later. He might have hit sooner, but after two murders, most middle-aged women in Cincinnati had become more than slightly cautious. Not Mrs. Jeanette Messer, however, a diminutive fifty-five-year-old woman who lived near the other victims. She not only continued to walk her dog alone in the woods early each morning, but she left the door of her home unlocked when she went out. At six-fifteen on the morning of June 10, 1966, a dog walker found her lying in the park. He thought she was a drunk sleeping it off. When he came upon two policemen a short while later, he reported the "bum sleeping in his underwear." When they went to check, they found Mrs. Messer. They didn't know at first who she was since her purse had been stolen, but the killer had tied Mrs. Messer's small black and white fox terrier, Judy, to a tree, and the police ultimately traced her identity through the dog tag.

Again they consulted Dr. Cleveland. By now he knew almost in advance what he would find, but he examined the situation carefully nonetheless. He saw that almost every bit of clothing had been ripped off her body, that she had been severely beaten around her face and head, and based on the size of each bruise, he established that the weapon, which was never found, was about two inches by four inches. He found that both of her cheekbones had been fractured by blows and surmised that she probably was never able to offer any resistance. He noticed that her ribs had been caved in, which meant that the killer either jumped or knelt on her. He noted that the blood and bent grass showed that she had been dragged about forty feet, at which time she either lost her shoes or had them removed by the killer. She was strangled with a dark blue and red paisley necktie found around her neck, and raped either after she died or while she was dying. Again he found pubic hairs, this time in a large quantity, and when the killer was found, he knew it would be easy to compare samples.

Otherwise, there were few clues. The tie used to strangle her was inexpensive and in no way distinctive. It could not be traced. A two-toned brown-and-white car had been seen parked near the murder site early that morning, but the year, make, or model was unknown. The police received hundreds of tips, and with nothing else to work on checked almost all of them, refusing however, the help offered by three clairvoyants. (Such help was accepted in the Boston Strangler case.) They were forced to check such calls as the one by a woman reporting the sinister way her neighbor walked, or another reporting that a man was cruising his car slowly down a street while a woman on the same street was walking her dog. (The man turned out to be recharging his battery.) The police also converged on a bar when they got a call that a man was discussing the crimes there—although the people of Cincinnati were beginning to talk of little else.

By now there was a run on tear-gas pens and door locks, but oddly enough, the latest killing increased, not decreased, the use of the woods near the University of Cincinnati. *The Cincinnati Enquirer* reported that the area was "strangled by sightseers," for thousands made a pilgrimage to see where Mrs. Messer had been killed. Probably no one checked the site out alone at six-fourteen in the morning.

Two months later another murder occurred. On August 14, 1966, Barbara Bowman, a thirty-one-year-old woman, was found lying in the street on a manhole cover, apparently the victim of a hit-and-run car. Miss Bowman was almost dead when they brought her into the hospital on that rainy morning, and she never lived to make it to the operating room.

When her body was brought to Dr. Cleveland later that day, he was relieved to hear that at least this time he did not have to work on another victim of the strangler, for the report in front of him stated that Bowman had been killed by a hit-and-run vehicle. But like all medical detectives, Cleveland let the body tell its own story.

In one hand she clutched a five-dollar bill. Dr. Cleveland noticed that she had a compound fracture of her right leg in two places, that her foot had been nearly severed at the right ankle, and that she had contusions and lacerations on the scalp and body. This was consistent with being hit by a car. But when he examined her neck, he was surprised to find a faint depression there, as if someone had tried to strangle her with an object such as a rope. Most people who accidentally run over someone do not first try to strangle her to death. Then Cleveland turned over the body and discovered something even stranger. She had been stabbed in the neck six times. In fact, he determined that it was the loss of blood from these wounds—not being run over—that was the real cause of her death.

Although her dress was pulled up to her waist and her shoes were off when she was found, Barbara had not been raped as were the first three victims of the strangler. Cleveland believes that her attacker may have tried to assault her sexually and failed, as she, being stronger than the other women, had put up a fierce fight.

Since it was now suspected that her death was homicidal, and not accidental, the police returned to the place where she had been found. There they found one of her earrings, her broken glasses, beads from her necklace, and her bloody shoes, showing that there obviously had been a struggle. A disabled taxicab was found nearby, and the blood on the radiator showed that this was the car responsible for the hit-and-run, which was beginning to look less and less like an accident. When the police examined the back seat of the cab, they found strands of Barbara's brown hair as well as beads from her necklace, meaning she had been *in* the car as well as hit by it.

Nearby, the police found a three-foot-long fuzzy rope with beads from Barbara's necklace still embedded in it, which Cleveland later established matched the depression on her neck. Twelve to fifteen feet away was a bloody paring knife. Based on the size of the stab wounds, Dr. Cleveland concluded that it might have been the murder weapon. This is not as simple to establish as it would seem, for the size of a wound is not the same as the size of the knife which produced it, and the same is also true for bullet wounds. The width of a knife wound is usually *less* than the width of the knife that caused it, because the skin is elastic and tries to return to its original size after it has been penetrated. In addition, in certain areas, the depth of the wound may be deeper than the length of the knife itself, because the soft tissue depresses as the knife enters.

What all this evidence told about the crime was chilling, for Barbara Bowman must have fought off three different attempts to kill her (a rope, a car, and a knife) before finally losing her battle. And she was not the type of girl who normally fought. She was a typist, about five feet, four inches tall, 110 pounds, with brown and frosted hair styled and teased around a pleasant face. She did not have the kind of looks that would make a man do a double-take, or perhaps even a single one, but she was known to be a sweet, quiet girl. She lived alone in a one-room apartment, went out rarely, and then mostly with girlfriends, attended church twice a week, woke up each morning at six-thirty to get to work, and paid her bills promptly. At the time of her death she was saving up for a vacation, and foolishly was carrying the money with her in her purse.

At seven o'clock on the final night of her life, she had a drink with a neighbor, and then went out with a girlfriend and the girl's boyfriend. The three went to the Lark Cafe—a few blocks from where Mrs. Messer had been killed. At about one in the morning, while her two friends decided to stay on, Barbara decided to go home so she could get up early for church the next day. Barbara then called for a cab—a rare, financial splurge for her before the strangler scare, but now almost a necessity, for most women in Cincinnati were too frightened to walk alone.

She called Cincinnati's Yellow Taxicab Company. A yellow taxicab came to pick her up, but what she did not know was that the driver was not employed by that company. He had stolen the cab from their lot that evening and had been radioing back and forth as if he was a legitimate driver, intercepting calls that rainy night, picking up customers, and pocketing whatever money he made. The pattern of his actions was later pieced together.

Earning a few dollars in this manner was probably all he had in mind that night, and most likely he started to take Barbara to her destination as he had done with his earlier customers. But two blocks from her home (where she was ultimately found), she must have taken out her money to pay him. Perhaps he spotted her vacation money and suddenly entered upon a robbery which ultimately became a murder.

In that heavily wooded area near her home, he must have tried to strangle her with the fuzzy rope, and failed because she was protected by the bead necklace. She managed to escape from the cab and fled while he probably attempted to run her down with the cab, then jumped out and stabbed her in the throat, leaving her to die in the rain on a manhole cover of a storm sewer.

There were many more clues in this murder than in the others, although the rain had obliterated all finger- or footprints. Even so, the killer was seen by more than one person. First, several customers at the Lark Cafe had seen him when he came to pick up Miss Bowman. Unfortunately, no one had taken a careful look at the man assumed to be just another cabbie. Secondly, he had been driven by another cab driver at around three o'clock that morning, shortly after the attack on Barbara Bowman. Another taxi driver had picked up a man in the area who hailed him by waving two rain-soaked one-dollar bills, later believed to have come from Barbara's purse. The real cab driver noticed that his passenger seemed nervous and out of breath, and made *him* nervous by constantly leaning over and breathing down his neck. When a police car passed, the passenger threw the wet bills at the driver and jumped out of the cab.

Another clue, and an important one, was that the murderer had a key that fit the ignition of all Yellow cabs, and he also knew how to operate taxis. He had picked up eleven fares before Miss Bowman and registered them on the meter. The killer apparently knew how to "sharp shoot" (intercept a call for a cab), and "short stop" (call in and give a false cab number), all of which meant that he probably had once been a cab driver, most likely for the Yellow Cab Company. In addition, therefore, to a clear description of the killer, the police now knew one of his former occupations—which unfortunately gave them about 5,000 people to check on. Still, with so many clues, it seemed obvious that the Cincinnati Strangler, as he was now being called in the papers (even though Bowman's killer may not have been he), was about to be caught.

The next time the people of Cincinnati heard about the strangler, it was not his name. Two months after Barbara Bowman's death, and one year after the first attack, another middle-aged woman, Mrs. Alice Hochhausler, fifty-one, was found strangled and raped. Not only did Mrs. Hochhausler meet her death by the strangler, but like Barbara Bowman she was killed because of her concern about him. Most of the women in Cincinnati were worried about him, but until Barbara Bowman was killed, it was only the older women who really feared for their safety. Now that a woman in her early thirties had died, almost no one felt safe anymore. But Mrs. Hochhausler's concern was mostly for one of her nine children, an attractive twenty-two-year-old nurse who worked one night a week at a local hospital. Mrs. Hochhausler, not wanting her daughter to ride in a taxi at night after the Barbara Bowman incident, would throw a trenchcoat over her bathrobe and pick up her daughter at the hospital. On that night, the mother drove her daughter home before midnight and then continued on to her own two-and-one-half-story brick house near Burnette Woods, the same woods where Mrs. Messer had been killed. Mrs. Hochhausler never made it home.

That night her husband, a surgeon, locked the family police dog, Rex, in the basement and fell asleep before his wife left to pick up their daughter. When he awoke the next morning and saw that his wife was not in bed, he went to the garage to see if the car was there. As he walked toward the garage, he came upon her possessions: one sneaker, her dentures, and finally her car keys. He found her lying in the driveway next to the car with her trenchcoat off, the cord of her red bathrobe around her neck, and her nightclothes in disarray.

Dr. Cleveland arrived at the scene at eight-thirty in the morning. He thought that as she had walked toward her home from the car that previous night, she probably had been struck on the back of her head so hard that it knocked out her false teeth and rendered her unconscious. The way he could tell that she was probably unconscious during the rest of the attack was that she had no bruises typical of a struggle—bruises on a victim's arms, for example, may indicate that he was held down; wounds over the shoulder blades may mean that he was pinned to the ground. When a person is stabbed to death, the wounds provide clues: in-and-out knife thrusts in a small area indicate that the victim did not fight or resist; stab wounds in the arms or hands, called "defense wounds," indicate that the victim put up his arms to ward off the knife.

A "patterned bruise" the size of a thumb on Mrs. Hochhausler's foot indicated that she had been dragged from her car by the ankle and then killed. The bathrobe cord and not the blows on her head caused her death, and this was important, for it showed that this was again the work of the strangler. After all, anyone wanting to do away with a middle-aged woman in Cincinnati that year could have killed her, say, with a blow on her head, and then placed a cord around her neck to make it look like the strangler. Again Cleveland found the same black pubic hairs, and enough blood to establish the killer's blood type—and again, as in the other crimes, it was type O.

One strong clue emerged. Hochhausler's daughter reported that after her mother had driven her home, they parked outside of her house for a few minutes to talk. A black man driving a 1959 tan-and-white Chevrolet pulled up behind them, and the mother wondered aloud why the man was waiting there. When her daughter walked across the street to her house and turned around to wave her mother goodbye at the door, she noticed that the same Chevy had pulled around her mother's car and was starting to drive slowly on. A brown-and-white car had been seen at the woods when Mrs. Messer was killed. The same car had been seen when Mrs. Dant was killed, although only now did the police find out the year and make of the vehicle.

The police used an IBM computer to track down every 1959 Chevrolet registered in Hamilton County, a herculean task, since the cars were not listed according to color, and fifteen thousand automobiles of that year and make were registered. Each had to be checked out individually, and the police could only do about fifty a day. They also asked people to report all brown-and-white Chevies (one black man in such a car was stopped seven times in two days) and to report anybody who looked suspicious—which meant black. Naturally, racial problems arose. Innocent blacks constantly were stopped and questioned, and many white women who saw a black man on their streets did not think black was beautiful and ran to call the police. The situation became so volatile that the head of the local NAACP made a public announcement begging the strangler to turn himself in.

It produced no results, and fears mounted. More than a year had passed since the first woman had been killed and people had become as paranoid as they were cautious. Some of the department stores exploited their anxieties by handing out free whistles to women who came into their stores. The hardware and weapon stores could not keep up with the demand for locks, guns, and tear-gas pens. Many women stopped opening their doors even to the Avon lady, and some went out only in pairs on a buddy system. Even the relatively innocent holiday of Halloween was disrupted, for the trick-or-treating was rescheduled to daylight hours so that no woman would have to open her door at night. No one felt safe anymore—not even the blacks in Cincinnati, who were subject to the wrath of the whites. The fact that only one of them was guilty was often forgotten in the panic.

Two weeks after the Hochhausler murder, Mrs. Rose Winstel, eighty-one years old, was found raped and strangled in her bedroom. Because of her cataracts, she could barely see people even five feet in front of her, and in her fear of the strangler, she left her home only about once a month. It did not matter. The strangler came there. This was the first time that he had forced his way into an apartment, and he had simply ripped all of the chain locks off her door.

When Dr. Cleveland arrived, he found the victim partly under her bed with the cord of her heating pad wound tightly around her neck. She was nude, her clothing in disarray underneath her body. She too had been raped, severely beaten around the head and neck with a blunt instrument, and dragged out of her bed. Cleveland noticed that there were more physical injuries here than on the other victims, and when this was reported in the papers, it made the women of Cincinnati even more nervous, worrying that the strangler—if there was only one—was becoming more violent with each crime.

Finally, six weeks later on December 9, 1966, the last victim was found—and on the same day so was a killer. Miss Lulu Kerrick, eighty-one years old, was a small, frail, sickly woman who lived alone. She was killed in the elevator of her apartment building very early in the morning, and when Dr. Cleveland arrived, he found her stockings knotted around her neck, her dress disarrayed, her dentures on the floor, her shoes removed, and her keys still in her hand. It certainly looked like the strangler-rapist again, although when he examined her body later in his office, he was surprised to discover that this time there were no black hairs—and she had not been raped. Nonetheless, Dr. Cleveland felt that the rest of the attack matched the pattern of the other murders and was therefore probably the work of the strangler. He had noticed a bright orange stain in Mrs. Kerrick's underpants, which is the result of taking a pill called pyridium. He wondered if the killer had started to rape her and on seeing the discharge become frightened or superstitious and not completed his act.

The news of this murder, however, was overshadowed by the news of the apprehension of a man charged with one of the murders. He was Posteal Laskey, a twenty-nine-year-old laborer and part-time guitarist in a jazz combo called The Outlaws. He had a police record which included allegations of attacks on two women; the first arrest had occurred three days before the first woman in Cincinnati had been attacked. Laskey had been imprisoned once for robbing a woman, and had been placed on three years' probation in October of 1965, the exact month in which the first attempted murder took place—after having been convicted on an assault and battery charge for beating up a woman he had followed home. Laskey had been questioned months earlier in conjunction with the Cincinnati stranglings and been released.

The police also found two strong pieces of circumstantial evidence against Laskey. It seems he had been a cab driver for six months for the Yellow Taxicab Company with the call number 186, and he had failed to turn in his key when he left. Furthermore, when Barbara Bowman's bogus cab driver had picked her up at the Lark Cafe, he had used the call number 186.

At first Laskey was not held for any of the murders in Cincinnati, but rather in connection with an incident that had occurred at twelve-thirty on the morning of Miss Lulu Kerrick's killing. At that time, a twenty-two-year-old woman, Mrs. Sandra Chapas, had been followed down the street and into her apartment building by a man she later claimed was Laskey. The man was frightened away by a neighbor just returning from work. Seeing a black man jump into a car—a cream-and-brown car—the man took down the license plate number and immediately reported it to the police. During the night the police traced the car to Laskey, and at five o'clock in the morning, several policemen converged on his home. Laskey, however, was not there, which gave them something to think about when they later learned from Dr. Cleveland that the time of Lulu Kerrick's death was about one hour later.

Six of the people who had been in the Lark Cafe on the night that Barbara Bowman was killed tentatively identified Laskey out of a police line-up of five men—although it was four months since the night of the Bowman murder, and none had had more than a fleeting glance at the cabdriver that night in the cafe. In addition, when Laskey's picture appeared in *The Cincinnati Enquirer*, a forty-five-year-old woman went to the police station and positively identified Posteal Laskey as the man who had recently attacked her while she was working in a church.

The woman claimed that Laskey had entered the church and asked where he could find the custodian. The woman said he could be found in the basement, but the man requested that she go with him. When she refused, he lunged at her neck, warned her not to make any sounds or he'd slit her throat, and threatened her repeatedly, ominously suggesting what must have been terrifying to a woman who had read of six murder-rapes in that area: "Do you want what the others got?" He then hit her twice, knocked her down, and was starting to choke her when the custodian entered. He knocked the custodian down cold with one blow, grabbed the woman's purse, and ran.

Laskey was not charged with all the murders. The Cincinnati police charged him with the first-degree murder of Barbara Bowman, larceny (of the taxi), and "assault" on Mrs. Chapas, though Laskey never physically touched her. (The charge was possible because the *elements* of assault—ability to inflict injury or fear—were present.) At his trial—which attracted only about twenty-five spectators despite all of the attention the murders had received—Laskey was well dressed and carried a book titled *How to Play Winning Chess.* With an all-white jury, it looked like the only thing Laskey would win.

Posteal Laskey claimed that he had been picked up by a friend on the evening of Barbara Bowman's death, and that the two had gone to the Soul Lounge together. He stayed until one or one-fifteen A.M. (Barbara's cab driver picked her up at about one and had driven eleven fares earlier) and arrived home at one-thirty or one-forty-five A.M. He did not go out again until he awoke the next morning at eight, he said. Various family members and friends said they had seen him home after one-thirty, and some of them testified that his clothes were not mud-splattered, bloody, or wet on that dismal rainy night.

Only one witness said she saw Barbara Bowman and Laskey together, for while those in the Lark Cafe had seen her with her friends, and others had seen him come in and shout "Cab," no one had seen the two leave together. But one witness came forth and said that at two-twenty on the morning of Barbara Bowman's death, she had pulled her car alongside a taxi to ask the driver for directions. No one was in the front seat, but as she shouted her question into the cab, Laskey raised himself up from the back seat, climbed over to the front, and got behind the wheel. It was at that point that she saw a girl in the back seat slowly rise up and then suddenly slump over as if something was wrong with her. What shocked the witness and made her remember it was the realization that the girl was white while the driver was black.

The defense tried to prove mistaken identity, and some of the testimony in the trial centered around Laskey's appearance. Although all of the customers at the Lark who had seen the cab driver gave the police a description of a man who looked like Laskey, and all identified him later in a police line-up, none mentioned that the man had a small goatee. He had not grown it since the murder, for witnesses were called in who testified that he had sported a beard for more than seven years. As the prosecution pointed out in court, however, it was hard to see the goatee when facing him head on.

The witnesses gave varying accounts of what he had been wearing that night, and there was considerable controversy over whether he had been wearing a peaked cap, as some said, or had no head covering, as others claimed. That he may have removed his cap at different times in the evening did not seem to be considered.

After eight hours of deliberation, the jury of six men and six women found Posteal Laskey guilty of the first-degree murder of Barbara Bowman and sentenced him to death. They did not recommend mercy. Although Laskey outwardly took his death sentence calmly, the black community of Cincinnati did not. Many blacks felt he had not received a fair trial and they did not fail to note that an all-white jury had convicted a black defendant of killing a white woman.

Actually, three blacks had been called as jurors, but all were excused—two on challenges by the prosecution, and one by the defense. It was also true, as the black community complained, that all of Laskey's defense witnesses were black, and none were believed, but of the prosecution witnesses, against Laskey, only two were black.

A drive began in the black community to raise funds for an appeal. Posteal Laskey's cousin, Peter Frakas, who had helped raise money for Laskey's legal defense, was frequently seen in Cincinnati carrying sandwich signs proclaiming "Laskey is innocent; Cincinnati is guilty." He was not exactly well-liked by the police department—which had spent hundreds of hours on this case and was constantly berated for not solving it quickly. At twelve-thirty-five A.M. Frakas was arrested on loitering charges for "blocking pedestrian traffic." According to the U.S. Riot Commission report the arrest set off a chain of events precipitating the riots that resulted in one death, sixty-three injuries, 404 arrests (85 percent of them black) and three million dollars in damage.

Meanwhile, Posteal Laskey, unaware that he had

become such a cause célèbre, sat in death row and received stay after stay of execution. He became the lead guitarist of the Ohio Penitentiary band, and his lawyer commented that an "electric guitar was the closest thing electric he'd ever get to." The Supreme Court decision against capital punishment proved him correct, and Posteal Laskey remains today in jail. And from the day he was jailed, no further rape-stranglings of this sort occurred in Cincinnati.

Some in Cincinnati say that Laskey killed only Barbara Bowman. Some believe he was responsible for all six deaths and that he was tried for the one murder alone because there was more evidence in the form of witnesses. Dr. Cleveland says: "They used their best case. There's other information that can't be released now but if they ever have to try him again they'll use it." The chances are that there will be no second trial, but if Dr. Cleveland had not had the curiosity to question whether "accidental hit-and-run" death might not be murder, Posteal Laskey would have gone free—and perhaps other women in Cincinnati might now be dead.

6

Disguising the Deceased: The Chemist and the Crusader

Charles Henry Schwartz was a good-looking young fellow in his early thirties who dressed well, spoke well, lived well, and was liked by everyone who met him. Schwartz had settled in Berkeley, California, after leaving the East, and while he was never specific when asked where he had lived before, he never failed to mention that he had spent a good deal of time overseas in the air force. He more than just mentioned it in passing. At parties he inevitably became the center of attention as he regaled his friends and acquaintances with colorful stories of his dramatic military exploits.

Schwartz was an accomplished raconteur and knew enough not to let his war stories get bogged down in minutiae. Instead, he would talk for hours in general terms about his amazing experiences as a flying ace who had been shot out of the sky on a dozen occasions. Of course, he invariably survived each crisis, though he was not loathe to admit that once his incredible luck almost failed him. On that occasion, *he* was shot instead of his plane and bailed out, almost dead; he added that he still had a scar on his chest from the original wound. Because of the lack of explicit dates and places in his stories, some of his friends thought that he might have been a spy, and since Schwartz neither denied nor confirmed the question, he thereby fanned the rumors.

When he settled down in California, rather than looking for a job in aviation, where he had had so much experience, he returned to the field of chemistry, which had been an interest of his before he entered the service. He had no trouble finding a job with a large chemical company, but he soon became bored with corporate anonymity and started thinking about ways to fly high on his own again. And so on the side in his spare time, he began working on a series of chemistry experiments.

Schwartz was a bright and capable scientist, and no one was surprised when after several weeks he announced dramatically that he had just discovered a way to produce an artificial silk that looked better and cost less than real silk. To support his statements, he had made a sample of his silk which not even experts could distinguish from the real product. Everyone was impressed and agreed his discovery had enormous potential. So he left his lowly lackluster job with the chemical company, found some financial backing, and started his own chemical company. A good deal of his financial support came from his wife, who until then had kept her own healthy bank account separate from his. With her help, and that of others, Schwartz built an impressive-looking factory and stocked it with all of the chemical equipment he would need in order to make his product a success.

Those who did not really know Schwartz or his invention thought that he had become wealthy already, although the truth was that he had not yet figured out how to mass produce his inexpensive silk and profitably put it on the market. So confident was he, however, of being able to overcome this problem that with the money left over after he had purchased the factory, he took out a mortgage on an expensive house in one of the better sections of Berkeley, and settled his wife and three children there. Although he seemed to be an open person, when his family and friends asked him for details about his invention, he became very secretive. No one knew whether he discussed the business aspects of his life with his closest friend, Gilbert Warren Berbe. But many things about the relationship between the two men were a mystery, and the most perplexing question was why Schwartz would have chosen to become friendly in the first place with a man like Berbe.

Gilbert Warren Berbe appeared to be the antithesis of Schwartz. While it was true that Berbe had also fought in the war, he did not sit around later and tell stories of his exciting experiences. Berbe returned a totally disillusioned man. Schwartz may have viewed the war as a stage for heroes; Berbe saw it as a game for fools. He brooded constantly about the death and devastation of war, and the year before he and Schwartz became close friends, he decided to do something about it. He was going to become a crusader.

Berbe relinquished all of his possessions, substituted patched-up rags for his button-down shirts, gave up his house to move into a dilapidated shack in the outskirts of the town, and gave away all of his money to the poor. He saved only a few dollars, just enough to buy a Bible, and his one self-indulgence was to have his name inscribed in gold on the flyleaf. Unlike some self-styled preachers or prophets, however, Berbe really did try to help others more than himself. He went around collecting money for the poor, comforting the blind and crippled, and giving solace to all who seemed in need. Naturally, everyone thought he was odd, but he was tolerated nonetheless and, because of his sincerity, well liked.

Suddenly—no one knew exactly when—Gilbert Berbe disappeared. His disappearance was not noticed immediately. Not even Schwartz mentioned it—and if the people of Berkeley gave it any thought, they assumed that he had holed up in his shack for a few days, or perhaps had left town. It is not uncommon for a peripatetic preacher to spread the word of God, and when interest and free food runs out, to run out himself. People knew that Berbe would eventually leave Berkeley, for he had often said that his mission was to cross the entire United States and make every inhabitant he met a happier person when he left him.

So when Berbe and his Bible disappeared from Berkeley, no one was surprised—or concerned. But a month later the townspeople began to talk about Berbe quite a bit, wondering whether he had really left Berkeley, and if so, how far away he had gone. The reason for this sudden interest was that something happened to Schwartz. One evening Schwartz remained at his factory working until late, dismissed the night watchman (an unusual act), and then called his wife to say he was on his way home. Schwartz never lived to keep that promise.

Five minutes after he placed that call to her, his entire factory, and everything in it—including Schwartz—went up in flames. The explosion was heard for miles. When the chief of the Fire Department examined what was left of the factory, he concluded that the explosion definitely was not an accident, for he found six torches surrounded with flammable materials, plus several powerful explosives against the wall, which had failed to ignite. The fire chief said that had they gone off, they would have lifted the entire building off the ground, and nothing whatsoever would have remained of Charles H. Schwartz to examine. While his body was severely burned, however, enough still remained to enable his wife (who was completely hysterical) and the night watchman (who was calm) to identify the body.

Almost nothing is known about the medical detective who performed the unpleasant autopsy, except that he had a Ph.D. in chemistry and obviously knew what he was doing. So badly burned was Schwartz's body that he was not surprised at finding no trace of the scar he had been told was over Schwartz's heart. But he was surprised to find that not all of the burns on Schwartz were uniform, and that some of them could not have been the result of the fire. His suspicions were confirmed when he saw through a magnifying glass that Schwartz's fingertips had been burned with some kind of acid. Another strange thing: Schwartz's eyes had been gouged out, hardly the effect of flames. It almost seemed as if someone knew Schwartz was going to be in that fire, and was trying to make certain that no one would ever be able to identify him. This obviously was not the simple case that it seemed. The medical detective decided to examine the body in more detail.

It did not take long for him to discover that Schwartz apparently had sustained a severe blow to the back of his head: he wondered whether the blow—and not the fire—was the real cause of death. If so, then Schwartz must have been killed *before* the fire started.

To determine if this was true he examined the mouth for soot and the blood for carbon monoxide. If a person is alive and breathing when a fire starts, he would breathe in the carbon monoxide and soot from the fire, and these will later be found in his body. If none is present, then the person was dead when the fire began. One exception has appeared in the last decade: when the victim is doused with gasoline and then set aflame (usually in gangland killings) or in cases of self-immolation (such as in protest against the Vietnam War). In this case death occurs so quickly that the person never has a chance to breathe in the products of the fire. But such was not the case with this chemical factory fire, and since Schwartz had no carbon monoxide in his blood or soot in his air passages the medical detective concluded that he died before the explosion occurred. Furthermore, the most likely cause of his death, the what-done-it, was that blow on the back of his head.

The night watchman, who had left the chemical factory twenty minutes before the explosion occurred, was suspected first. But he immediately tried to make it look as if it were Schwartz, and not he, who had acted suspiciously that evening. He said that when he had brought Schwartz some soup for dinner that night, he had noticed that his employer looked worried and nervous. He did not attach any importance to it at the time, because he had often noticed that Schwartz was like that when completing each stage of his experiments. The watchman said he had not even wanted to leave the factory that night, but Schwartz had given him some money and told him to buy an alarm clock and chewing gum. Furthermore, he specifically told him not to hurry back but to take a couple of hours off, and find something to do. Because it was late, however, and the watchman had no place to go, he returned to the factory within the half-hour. Schwartz had flown into a fury. He insisted the watchman leave immediately. This he did with some relief, for, as he told the police, Schwartz had been acting strangely all day. For example, he said, Schwartz had a secret closet under the stairs, and he kept looking at it nervously all that day. When the watchman's dog had stopped and scratched at the closet door that afternoon, Schwartz had leaped up and violently lost his temper.

The police decided to check the contents of the cupboard to see whether the watchman was telling the truth when he intimated that Schwartz had something to hide. The closet was empty, but when the police inspected it closely they found what looked like traces of dried blood. As they were starting to examine that, deep in the corner of the closet they spotted something else. It was a Bible, with the name of Gilbert Warren Berbe inscribed in gold on it. The police asked the medical detective to examine the burned body again to see if it really was Schwartz.

Or Berbe.

Identification of a murder victim is often hindered by deliberate dismemberment or disfigurement. Whoever killed the man in the chemical plant had gouged out his eyes and burned off his fingertips, although as it turned out this was a mistake, for it only aroused the suspicions of the police. Someone wanted to disguise Schwartz's identity. (The usual assumption, when fingerprints are found to have been removed, is that the victim had a criminal record with fingerprints on file. The police then try to identify the *face* of the person with police photographs rather than his fingerprints.)

Murderers who do not want their victims known by a tattoo may remove that as well. But often the medical detectives can tell the victim did have a tattoo at one time, although of course they cannot tell what it said. Tattoos are made by imbedding pigment in the layers of the skin; after a while the pigment becomes absorbed in the body and deposited in the person's lymph glands. The medical detectives in checking the lymph glands have one more clue to the identity of the deceased.

Clothing often tells the medical detectives something about the dead man. The clothing sometimes carries the name of the store in which it was purchased; it reflects the person's financial status. Or it may contain laundry marks that enable the police to identify the victim. Once a laundry mark was found on an unidentified man's shirt, but when the police tracked it down, they found the shirt belonged to someone who was very much alive. It seemed that the shirt belonged to the dead man's partner, who was so cheap that he would slip his clothes into the other's laundry to get them done for free.

The manner in which the deceased was dressed once told the medical detectives the what-done-it. When a group of air-raid victims was brought into an English mortuary and undressed, the pathologist noticed that one of the women's underpants were on inside out. He decided that something must have happened—and her pants hastily put on. He looked for signs of a recent abortion, and his suspicion was correct. The abortionist had apparently placed her dead body with legitimate air-raid victims to make her death seem like it came from the bombing.

Many murderers do more than merely remove fingertips, tattoos, or clothes. The all-time record must be awarded to the husband who dismembered his wife, baked her head, and then painted it green so that no one could see who she was. The medical detective, Dr. John Devlin, deputy chief medical examiner of New York City, figured it out anyway. He noticed that she had marks on her skin characteristic of a "skin popper," or someone who injects heroin under the skin. Since most female junkies have to turn to prostitution, and many prostitutes have police records, he turned her fingerprints over to the police, who identified her.

One of the strangest cases of dismemberment was done not for criminal purposes but for so-called scientific ones. Franz Joseph Haydn may be best known for his *Surprise* Symphony, but the greatest surprise may have come at his own end. He died in 1809 during the height of a pseudo-science called phrenology, which taught that various talents and inclinations were controlled by certain "faculties" in our skull. One phrenologist who sought to find the faculty of music removed Haydn's head from his grave. After he examined the skull, pompously proclaiming that Haydn had a very well-developed "bump of music," he gave it to a woman who conducted musical soirées and who for eleven years garishly displayed it in a glass case for her guests.

Meanwhile, the Prince of Austria decided to have Haydn reburied, and when the grave was opened, it was discovered that something was missing: the head. The Prince ordered whoever had the head to return it. The woman told her husband she would never comply. The husband was frightened of the Prince, but more petrified of his wife; so he obtained another skull from a morgue which was united with the rest of Haydn's lonely bones. Although the truth eventually came out, it was not until 1954 that Haydn's head was returned to the body to which it belonged.

Even when a body is not dismembered or mutilated, it is often difficult to identify. The medical detectives must concentrate on the unique aspects of the person they find. The results are often Sherlock Holmesish, whose author, incidentally, was a doctor and once studied under a medical detective. One medical detective saw that an unidentified man had an enlarged big toe—and correctly surmised that he may have been a ballet dancer. The identity of all missing male ballet dancers was checked, and the body soon known and named. In another case, a medical detective noticed calluses on an unidentified woman's knees. His first thought was that she was a washerwoman or maid, but then he saw that her hands were not rough. Who else spends much time on her knees, he wondered? A nun. Her description was matched with those of missing nuns and she was soon identified.

Some interesting work has been done on identification solely from stomach contents. A cab driver who despised his wife took her to a party and killed her on the way home. A body was found later, but the husband could not be prosecuted unless it proved to be his wife's. Lye had been used to destroy the body and the standard clues failed to reveal anything conclusive. Visual identification was impossible. Then the medical detectives examined her stomach contents and found traces of oranges, raisins, cherries, and almonds. The police visited the hostess of the party and asked her what she had served that night. "Let's see now," she said. "A fruit salad; I make it with oranges, cherries, almonds, and raisins." The husband was electrocuted.

Bones and teeth are among the best means of identification and they are likely to remain even if burned—as a janitor once found out after murdering someone and burning the body in his apartment house furnace. He had a lot of unexpected witnesses against him in court, because the residents of his building all testified that they remembered how hot it had been that night inasmuch as he had turned the heat up high to get rid of the teeth and bones.

Even when only a few bones are found, if they are the right bones, they can reveal much information about the person. A famous English pathologist, Sir Sidney Smith, was once brought two hip bones and a sacrum, in which a bullet was imbedded. He saw that together they formed a pelvis. He deduced that the deceased was female, for a woman's pelvis differs from a man's, being designed for childbearing. He deduced that she was short and light in weight and that her age was twenty-three or twenty-four, for the iliac bones had not yet fully fused with the pelvis as they would between the ages of twenty-two to twenty-five. And from a few pieces of soft tissue clinging to her bones, he deduced that she had died about three months earlier from septic peritonitis as a result of the bullet wound. Most important, her right hip bone, which was bigger and heavier than her left, from bearing most of her weight, indicated that she had a pronounced limp. From what he discovered from just three bones, the police had enough information to establish her identity and, ultimately, who killed her.

Just how much teeth can tell about an unidentified person is illustrated by the following story. In the 1960s a woman who had been strangled to death was found floating in a swamp in the northern part of Tokyo. At first glance, the medical detectives thought she was probably in her early twenties, but since they knew nothing else about her, they examined her teeth. Dental work varies geographically, and the first thing noticed was that her dental work had probably been done by an urban dentist, suggesting she lived in the city. But the medical investigators also noticed that the type of dental work she had done was for problems a woman of thirty-five to forty might have, and not a young girl. In addition, they saw that while she seemed to have taken good care of her teeth, the discolored roots and heavy tartar indicated a chain smoker. At that time in Japan, smoking was an extremely important clue, for only a woman who worked in a bar, cabaret, restaurant, or night club would be permitted to smoke so heavily that she could have obvious signs from it on her teeth. From these clues which came solely from her teeth, she was identified in six days. She was the forty-year-old proprietor of a Tokyo bar, killed by her co-proprietor, her lover.

While it has not yet been proven that teeth are as unique as fingerprints, their individuality in general is accepted, for the average person has thirty-two teeth, with five surfaces, each with its own peculiarities and differing further in arrangement, bite, arch, alignment, cavities, fillings, and even the dental repair work done on them. One dental detective, Dr. Lowell Levine, noticed that while an unidentified man's dental work had been carefully done, it was an amateurish job, suggesting to him that it might have been done by a dental student. The police checked dental students' records until they found records for their man.

Tracing unidentified people through teeth is facilitated because most dentists keep detailed records of their patients' teeth which can be matched with the teeth of the unidentified person. Even if the dentist does not keep records, he can often recognize his own work—as did Paul Revere, the silversmith and the first person in America to identify someone by his teeth. Although Revere is most famous today for his equestrian ride, he was actually the dentist who made George Washington's false teeth. He also made a dental bridge for a Dr. Joseph

Warren, who, killed at the Battle of Bunker Hill, was buried in a common grave. After the Revolution, the colonists wanted to honor Warren, but, unable to tell which body was his, called on Revere, who identified him by the bridge in his mouth.

Teeth are a good sign of age (especially of children since certain teeth appear at set times) and of habits. For example, heavy tartar and discoloration may show that the person smoked cigarettes; a characteristic V on a canine means that the person was a pipe smoker who wore that tooth down from holding the stem in the same place. Teeth also reflect the deceased's financial situation, for gold inlays and good dentures indicate high socioeconomic status, and unfilled cavities and unreplaced missing teeth usually suggest poverty (it can also be a sign of drug usage, since addicts neglect their teeth and heroin use leads to a craving for sweets).

The medical detective examining Schwartz's body had been told that Schwartz's teeth, despite his background, had become discolored, broken, and decayed, while Berbe, who had once been wealthy, had kept his teeth in excellent condition. So the first thing he examined was the teeth, and they were good. He had also been informed, however, that Schwartz was missing two teeth, and he noticed that two of this man's teeth were gone. It appeared the body, then, was Schwartz's. But how could it be explained that this man's teeth were good and Schwartz's were not? He examined the gums around the missing teeth and saw that they had not started to heal, meaning that the teeth had only recently been extracted. It seemed as if someone had deliberately gone out of his way to make it look like Schwartz was in the fire—but was he?

The medical detective could progress no further without a picture of Schwartz. The police asked Mrs. Schwartz for one, and she then told them of something that had occurred right after the fire that was so strange that she had felt it was too silly to report. But three days after the explosion someone had broken into the house and taken all the photographs, frames and all, of Schwartz; and nothing else. Since she remembered which studio had taken his professional portraits, the police simply had them reprinted from the original negatives in the files. Then they gave them to the medical detective.

Not much of the face of the man in the fire was left, but one crucial feature remained intact: his ears. Although to the layman all ears look pretty much alike, they have many distinctive features and next to friction ridges such as fingerprints, they are the most characteristic and unchangeable part of the body. Ears have occasionally played a part in solving crimes. For example, a Paris bank clerk once tried to disguise himself to abscond from France with the bank's money. He cut his bushy hair and dyed it gray, starved himself to lose weight, put irritant into his eyes to make them small and runny, pasted on false whiskers, puffed out his nose with a paraffin injection, and stooped over hobbling on a cane. He was caught the first time he ventured out of his house by a detective who had been shown his "before" photograph and knew enough to look out for the one feature that he could not alter—his ears. Ears have also unmasked imposters, and the woman who claimed to be the Grand Duchess Anastasia (upon whom the book, movie, and play were based) had a plausible story and a convincing manner, but her ear did not match that in the profile picture of the real daughter of Czar Nicholas. And here too, the ears of the man found in the fire did not match those in Schwartz's picture, for the deceased had a Darwinian tubercle on the outer lobe, and Schwartz did not. So Schwartz was definitely not the man in the fire.

The medical detective was able to acquire enough information from one badly burned body to tell that the man had been murdered before the fire started (examination of mouth and blood); most likely by a blow on his head (examination of the head); that the assailant had attempted to mask his victim's identity (gouging out the eyes, burning off the fingertips, and removing two teeth); that the victim had characteristics of Berbe (teeth), and could definitely not have been Schwartz (ears). The Bible in the cupboard and the sudden disappearance of its owner suggested that the man in the fire was probably Berbe, murdered by Schwartz in an elaborately staged murder scheme. The medical detective had solved practically every aspect of the crime with almost nothing to work on, but the motive to the murder remained for the police and regular detectives to solve.

Schwartz probably murdered Berbe not because he had anything against him, but because he had to kill someone and he knew Berbe's disappearance would cause no alarm. Leonard Gribble, who studied this case in detail, reports that Schwartz had first tried to find someone else to kill. Two or three weeks before the fire, he had advertised for a laboratory assistant. The advertisement contained the strange requirement that the applicant have small hands and feet, a requirement which made more sense once the police found out that Schwartz's appendages were almost effeminately small. Schwartz had even gone so far as to interview someone for the job, but for reasons that will never be known, ultimately chose Berbe as the victim.

Why would a respectable successful chemist on the

verge of making millions from a unique invention want to kill someone and blow up his own factory? Schwartz and his laboratory both turned out to be fakes. Charles Henry Schwartz, who was known earlier in other cities as Lester Henry Schwartz, and by the rather ridiculous John Doe Stein, was living a lie. He had never been a spy—at least not for our side. He *had* been in the war—but he had never even been in a plane. He had been the army unit barber. The so-called research laboratory that he had built had no gas, no water pipes, and not even a light in the main work room, so that the only available illumination came from an adjoining room. It would have been impossible for him to undertake serious research on his invention, as he claimed. Actually, his so-called secret formula turned out to have been copied from a manufacturing chemist's book, and the pieces of silk he showed around for demonstration purposes, which had supposedly been produced by his secret method, he had purchased for eight dollars.

Schwartz had built an impressive-looking laboratory, but when his backers, and especially his wife, wanted to see more for their money than promises, he was trapped. Insuring himself for $200,000 in case of accidental death, he hired someone to set fire to the place (he was eventually caught) and killed Berbe to put a body in the fire that could be confused with his. Since there were obvious dissimilarities, he gouged out the eyes, burnt off the fingerprints and removed two teeth. His last step was to put Berbe in the fire (he had probably been keeping his body in that secret closet) and disappear, hoping it would look as if he had been killed accidentally in the holocaust. And he would have gotten away with it, too, had the unignited explosives gone off, for then there would have been absolutely nothing left for the medical detective to examine. Had this happened, he would have continued with the rest of his plans, which were, as it turned out, to admit everything to his wife, who apparently knew nothing about his scheme, and hope that she would forgive him and share the insurance money he had worked so hard to get. But he never had the chance.

Although a search for him was immediately started, it was a while before two men came to the police with a promising lead. They said that they had rented a room in their boarding house to someone who looked like Schwartz, and who admitted that he was hiding out from the law over a minor problem. The boarder never left his room and never talked to anyone about anything—with one exception: the Schwartz case. This seemed to fascinate the boarder, who admitted that he knew something about chemistry, and said that the man in the fire could only have been Schwartz. The two men began to suspect their boarder's integrity, and the police concurred.

A group of policemen assembled outside of Schwartz's rooms in the lodging house and ordered him to open up the door. When he did not answer, they tried to break down the door. They failed on the first attempt, and as they were regrouping their forces to try again, they heard a pistol shot inside. At that moment, they broke down the door and saw in the front room a packed suitcase and some money, for Schwartz had apparently sensed trouble and was ready to flee. They also found a note to his wife confessing his guilt and begging for forgiveness for having hoodwinked her of all but $600 of her money.

In the other room lay Charles Henry Schwartz, dead from the bullet he had shot into his head.

7

Perfect Poison: The Horn & Hardart Mystery

A man and woman were found dead at a Horn & Hardart restaurant with cyanide of potassium in their stomachs. The woman was lying on the stairs leading to the mezzanine; the man was in the men's room. It seemed unlikely that the two had come into the restaurant together, for he looked like a neatly dressed businessman, while she was wearing filthy, patched-up rags. Furthermore, although the two lived in the same neighborhood near the restaurant, her "home" was the corner of an unused cellar whereas he lived in a respectable apartment. There seemed to be no relationship between these two people. Yet hypothesis of a suicide pact, or a suicide and murder, was not ruled out. There had to be some connection between the two, because cyanide of potassium is neither so common nor so accessible that each could have bought it independently and died from it at the same time and place. (It was ruled out that a third party could have poisoned them.)

Both of their backgrounds therefore had to be checked to see how and why they might have ingested the poison.

The man once had been a successful businessman, but had lost all his money. Now, at the age of fifty, he owed $150 in bank notes but had assets of only a few dollars. The woman, a frequent visitor to this restaurant, was a compulsive collector, and wore clothes patched together from garbage-can rags. In fact, her entire apartment looked like the rubble of a demolished building and was filled with everything she could find. She carried a shopping bag with her each day to help gather her collection, and when she was found dead that day, a half-eaten bread-roll filled with cyanide of potassium was still in her bag. How did the poison get into the two of them and was it a suicide pact, suicide and murder, suicide and accident, or accident and murder?

Poisoning, like most means of death, can be natural, accidental, suicidal, or homicidal. In the last category it can be very difficult to detect, because poisoners tend to be more intelligent than other murderers. As a result, not only may the poison they choose be undetectable or "perfect," but the manner in which they get the poison into their victims is often extremely clever. Several centuries ago, poisoners often settled for just dumping it into their victim's food or water, and such homicidal poisonings became so common that kings and members of their courts employed food and wine tasters as a precaution. (The reason the host currently tastes the wine first is to assure his guests that it's good enough for them, but the custom probably arose during the days when the host had to assure his guests that they too were not about to be poisoned.) Still, some of the early methods of getting poison into their victims were clever. It is said that in the fifteenth century, when a court physician decided to kill the King of Naples, he put the poison on the lips of his own daughter, the king's mistress, and waited for the king to kiss her.

In the twentieth century the methods have tended to be ingenious—in fact, the above method was used a few years ago to dispose not of a king but of a potential wife. A young man and his fiancée were found dead on the sofa the morning before their wedding with flushed faces and blood in their mouths. Cyanide was found in both of them, suggesting a suicide pact. It was later discovered, however, that the groom had gotten cold feet and decided to kill his bride rather than go through with the wedding. As he chewed gum a lot, he dosed his gum with poison and kissed her, intending to switch the gum into her mouth then. But underestimating its potency, he inadvertently swallowed some of the poison himself.

Another unique method of getting cyanide into a victim was devised by the Russians after World War II to kill some Ukrainian Nationalists. The K.G.B. agents put cyanide in a tube covered with a newspaper, pointed it at their victims and squeezed it. It all happened so quickly and so subtly that death was attributed to heart disease and no autopsies were ordered. The story was only known because a defecting agent revealed it.

One clever American dentist killed his father-in-law for his insurance by filling a cavity with aconitine or "monk's hood," a poison so deadly that one milligram, or 1/29,000th of an ounce, can be fatal. The dentist then covered it with a temporary filling which, coming out during the night, killed the father-in-law. The medical detective became suspicious when he found undissolved dental wax in the stomach. He started an investigation which led to the conviction of the dentist. (There were rumors during World War II that leading members of the Third Reich had placed poison in their teeth caps so that they could quickly commit suicide if caught. If true, it was probably either aconitine or nicotine.)

Possibly the most bizarre method of poisoning, although not the best since it was easily detected, was invented two centuries ago by a man who murdered five of his six wives. He got the poison into them during love-making. The first time, he wrapped a large amount of arsenic in a thin piece of paper, placed it up against the head of his penis, had intercourse, and waited for the poison to be absorbed through the vaginal walls. With another wife, he inserted the arsenic with his fingers, a process modestly described in the 1786 Criminal Archives as, "he placed two fingers into her vagina and thus tickled her for the time taken in saying two or three 'Our Fathers.' " By the time he got to his sixth wife, or she had gotten to him, he combined the two methods, inserted the arsenic with his fingers, and immediately had intercourse with her twice to push the paper up high. When he finally was caught he was sentenced to life imprisonment, chained to a cell wall and fed only bread and water. In addition he was branded on both sides of his face and received fifty strokes in the marketplace plus twenty-five more for every month of his life.

People are occasionally poisoned by accident, and different jobs have their own special hazards. Occupational poisoning has existed for centuries and has even become part of our vocabulary and literature. The expression "mad as a hatter" (like the Mad Hatter in Carroll's *Alice in Wonderland*) is said to derive from the bizarre behavior which results from mercury poisoning, a common hazard among hatmakers who used mercury in making felt hats.

Homicidal poisoning also sometimes can be accidental, which does not mean that a person did not plan a crime, but that he did not plan to kill with his poison. This occasionally occurs when criminals use chloroform to silence their victims, sometimes accidentally silencing them forever. In one case, however, a man accidentally poisoned a woman not to quiet her but to excite her—sexually, that is. The poison was cantharides, also known as "Spanish fly," which in small quantities acts as an aphrodisiac that causes repeated orgasms. In fact, the early medical literature reports the case of a man who took a "love potion" spiked with cantharides and then approached his wife eighty-seven times that night. Not surprisingly, he died the next morning. What happened to his wife was not recorded.

But cantharides is as potent as it makes the men who take it, and is a very dangerous poison with no known antidote. The Englishman who used the poison as an aphrodisiac stuffed it in some chocolate-covered coconut ice cream and then gave it to two girls in his office, thus causing their deaths. He later admitted that he had been in love with one of them, a twenty-seven-year-old brunette, and that he had made love with her about three months before. When he tried to repeat his performance, however, she had rebuffed him. He then hit upon this plan to make her more amorous, and another girl unwittingly ate the ice cream as well. He received five years' imprisonment for manslaughter. A similar situation occurred with the Marquis de Sade, and the poison was also cantharides. But instead of manslaughter he was charged with debauchery and fined the equivalent of $100.

The medical detectives in this field (called toxicologists, and usually Ph.D.s rather than M.D.s) have to figure out not just how the poison got into their victims—their main job is to figure out *what* poison. Just as the way that poisons are secretly administered has become increasingly sophisticated, so have the poisons. The result has been a race between murderers who have discovered new poisons, and the medical detectives who must stay one step ahead and figure out how to detect them in the victims' bodies. Not only are doctors often the toxicologists who catch poisoners, but, not surprisingly, many of the poisoners are often doctors or connected with the medical profession. (One argument against Sam Sheppard's having killed his wife was that, as a doctor of osteopathy, he could have found more subtle methods of dispatching her than bludgeoning her to death.)

It was a doctor who came up with what may be the nearest thing to a perfect murder, although he did not do it with poison—just words. This middle-aged surgeon fell in love with a young girl but could not marry her because his wife would not give him a divorce. One day his wife told him that she had a lump on her breast, and although he suspected what it probably was, he did not tell her about it. Instead, he reminded her that she had been thinking about taking a three-month European vacation and suggested that this was a good time for it. He left her with instructions to massage her breast for five minutes each morning and five minutes each night. When she returned, the lump was larger, "fixed" to the underlying tissue, and the cancer was too far gone to save her life.

In the old days it did not take a doctor to figure out which poison had been administered: it was usually arsenic, chosen because in some forms it is relatively tasteless, the signs and symptoms are similar to many natural diseases so that no suspicion is aroused, and it is relatively easy to acquire. But the reason why smart poisoners searched for something better was that arsenic does not disappear. Remains of it—usually in the hair and nails—can be found by the medical detectives centuries after the victim's death.

Arsenic cannot be destroyed by fire, or by cremating the poisoned person. Indeed, there is exactly as much arsenic today as there was in the beginning of time. But it is often hard to prove that someone deliberately gave his victim arsenic, because traces of the element can always be found in the human body. All of us eat it in minute quantities, and the Styrian arsenic eaters from Austria devour it with no ill effects or symptoms. Because arsenic is already in our bodies, and because some choose to ingest it in large quantities, the defense attorney in a poison trial usually implies that the arsenic got into the victim by natural means, or that he was secretly taking it on his own with great gusto like a secret alcoholic. But when *large* amounts of arsenic are found in the hair and nails it suggests it did not get there naturally. When arsenic enters the body, the organism first attempts to eliminate it, and then to render it harmless by absorbing or anchoring it in our hair and nails, which can absorb more arsenic without harm than other areas. Therefore, the quantity in the hair and nails is supposed to enable the medical detectives to determine when the poison was first administered, although this usually works out better in mystery books than in reality.

The arsenic in Napoleon's hair led Forshufuud, Smith, and Wassen, who studied all of Napoleon's ubiquitous ailments, to suggest that Napoleon may have died from acute and chronic arsenic poisoning. The cause of Napoleon's death has long been in doubt, although it is generally believed that he died from an extensive cancerous lesion of the stomach. The doctor who performed the autopsy thought he may have died from hepatitis. Still, in those days the symptoms of arsenic poisoning were not so well known as they are today.

Napoleon was extremely ill during the 100 days in 1815 after he escaped from Elba, and until his death he alternated between periods of relative health and extreme illness. His host of symptoms would take too much space to enumerate here, but many of them do correspond to arsenic poisoning. His autopsy report also suggested the same, as did the state of his body two decades after his death.

People who die from arsenic are often amazingly well-preserved. Although Napoleon was never embalmed, his body was well-preserved when his coffin was opened nineteen years after his death. Forshufuud, testing a hair from Napoleon's head, probably taken on the day after his death, found that it had 10.30 parts per million of arsenic, while the normal amount would be closer to 0.8 ppm. Napoleon himself thought he was being poisoned, and there is still dispute whether his words were simply paranoid prattling or whether he accidentally was being poisoned by medication—a phenomenon not uncommon in those days. Just before his death, he wrote in his will: "My death is premature. I have been assassinated by the English oligarchy and their hired murderer."

Poisoners today are usually too sophisticated to use arsenic, and choose other poisons in hopes of finding the "perfect" one. For a poison actually to be perfect, it should be tasteless, odorless, toxic, have no known antidote or delayed ill effects (so the murderer has time to cover his tracks); it should mimic the signs and symptoms of natural disease; and finally, it should be capable of administration without being obvious.

There are two exceptions to the rule of easy administration. One is in cases of infanticide, for the parents can force just about anything down the child's mouth. The other is revealed in the following unusual case. A host once became intoxicated after the party he threw, locked the door after his last guest left, and passed out. He woke up twenty minutes later with a violent burning in his throat and two days later he died. The poison found in his body was sulphuric acid, which works so quickly that the medical detective knew that he could not have taken it at the party without showing immediate signs from it. Neither could he have taken it before he slept, however, for then he would have been too ill to fall asleep. Since he was in the habit of sleeping with his mouth open, it turned out that his wife simply dropped it in while he was asleep.

One final—and crucial—quality of the perfect poison is that there should be no internal or external changes evident at the autopsy which the medical detectives could notice. According to Dr. Charles Umberger of the New York Medical Examiner's Office, the perfect way to poison someone would be to set up a container of carbon dioxide next to him while he was sleeping and remove the receptacle in which the dry ice was placed. It would take about thirty seconds for the person to die from anoxia (lack of oxygen) because the gas, being heavier than air, would settle down on the victim. Furthermore, it would leave no traces in the body.

Dr. Umberger believes that a great number of poisons today are perfect in the sense that the medical detectives would have a hard time finding one if they did not know in advance what to look for. He explains:

"Because of the changing nature of toxicology, our routine analysis would miss forty percent of the poison on the market right now. In 1940 there were only about sixty possible poisons that could kill, and they were all extracts of natural plant products. But in the nineteen fifties, the pharmaceutical houses found a synthetic way to make the same natural product; other houses changed the structure slightly, and soon there were ten variations of the same product. Other houses copied their formulas with minor variations, and the result today is perhaps 5,000 bases with 250,000 possibilities. Unless we know what we're looking for, there isn't enough tissue in the body to enable us to test for everything. In the old days, we'd turn to our books and test from A to Z till we found the poison. Today we can't get through the As."

Dr. Umberger explains that the reason most poisoners are caught is not just because of the toxicologists, but because the poisoners in some way tell the toxicologists what to look for. It is hard to get hold of a rare poison without detection and poisons are often needed in large quantities. Almost invariably, they feel a compulsion to discuss the "perfect poison" in public. Once the medical detectives have been told what to look for, they can find it. Another reason that poisoners are caught is that they are so flushed with success at eradicating one person that they often decide to repeat their achievement. In many instances it has been the number of deaths, not the type, that first aroused suspicion.

One of the most blatant examples of this occurred when a young wife decided to become a young widow. After killing her husband with poison, she discovered that her six children were keeping her from acquiring a new husband. So she killed them off, one by one, married a rich older man, and then killed *him* off. After that she married for love a man with four children, only to discover that she liked his four children about as much as she had liked her own six. She got around to killing off only two of them, before people started counting—and wondering.

The solution to the case of the woman who collected things and the down-and-out businessman is as follows: the man, burdened by his debts and seeing no other way out, decided to kill himself. He bought some cyanide, went to Horn & Hardart's, and got a bread-roll to make the poison more palatable. He put the cyanide into the bread, bit into it, put it down, and made it to the men's room before dying. A suicide.

The woman spent much of her time seated at the Horn & Hardart mezzanine, mesmerized by the people eating their meals below. When someone left without finishing his food, she would swoop down and grab it for her useless collection. But like most misers, she would eat some of the leftovers to save on her marketing bill. Thus she bit into that man's roll before dropping it in her shopping bag, and poisoned herself. So died two people with no relation to each other. By the way, this case had a strange twist. Author Richard Tobin reports that later the police found that this scavenger had accumulated more than $45,000 in various banks, which she never touched. By drawing on the interest alone, she could have paid that man's debts several times over and saved both lives.

PART III

BEYOND MURDER: SUICIDE, SEX, AND DRUGS

8

Suicide

A thirty-two-year-old married RAF officer fell in love with an attractive Welsh corporal, although fraternization was frowned upon by their superiors. When the girl's commanding officer found out about her affair, arrangements were made to have her transferred. According to her lover, who was the only one left to tell the story later, the two made a suicide pact. He said she first shot herself through the chest with his gun, then changed her mind and asked him to go for help. As he was leaving, he heard her fire the second fatal shot. He then lost the courage to keep his part of the bargain.

The medical detective who examined the body of the badly disfigured girl noticed the following: the wound in her left breast had bled copiously. Little blood, however, was lost from the massive head wound, and from the extent and location of the head wound, he knew that death must have resulted from it instantaneously. In addition, the bullet that was fired twelve to eighteen inches away from her head entered above her left eye and emerged over her right ear. And finally, when she was found, her left hand lay loosely across the wound in her left breast. Was it really a suicide or had her lover killed her?

Deciding whether a death is suicidal or homicidal is not always simple. Every method a person can use to commit suicide also can be used to kill him (with the exception of manual strangulation) and a person can be given a fatal dose of barbiturates, hung up to look like a suicide after he is murdered, or tossed out of the window as if he had jumped. So it is not always possible to establish whether death was homicidal or suicidal merely by examining the victim, for the circumstances surrounding the death and impinging upon the person at the time he chose to die—*if* he chose to die—must also be analyzed. While there are certain indications of suicide, there are just as many exceptions.

People often assume that a suicide note means the person killed himself. Actually, murderers have forced their victims to write suicide notes, and there is a good fictionalized example of something similar in Ira Levin's *A Kiss Before Dying*. In that story, a young man gives his victim a Spanish passage to translate, and later the despairing paragraph in the victim's handwriting is considered proof that she was depressed enough to kill herself.

In real life, classic suicide notes are sometimes found although the person died a natural death. Some seriously ill people decide not to wait for death and in a fit of depression write a suicide note and then change their minds. Since people rarely date their notes, confusion arises when these are found later after the person died a natural death.

For example, an old, badly-dressed man was once found with the following note in his pocket: "No money. No hoam. No famiely. Nobody. Thys wey best. Daeth last security. Am sorry." It turned out that his death came not from his own hands but from a heart attack. The note was soiled and the brown edges indicated it had been written long before his death at a time when, perhaps not surprisingly considering his circumstances, he was contemplating an end to his misery.

Of course, a death is more likely to be classified as suicide when the deceased is known to have threatened to kill himself. But many people talk of killing themselves without doing so. Furthermore, a potential suicide who is paranoid may project his suicidal impulses, insisting that others are trying to kill him. One woman, for example, told everyone in her neighborhood, including the chief of police, that her husband was trying to poison her. When she was found dead of poison, her husband was immediately suspected. He was saved only by the toxicological report which showed that she had died by swallowing an entire bottle of crude nicotine, a poison so strong and so vile that her husband never could have administered much of it to her without a struggle that would have left clues on the body.

Often, the death scene may contain clues that hint of homicide rather than suicide, such as forced entry or evidence of another person (food and drink for two or cigarette butts when the victim did not smoke). Signs of struggle, or the room and dead person in disarray, also suggest homicide, since suicides usually do not fight. They ordinarily do not shoot themselves more than once, either, except that occasionally they fire a "hesitation shot." In these cases, as they fire the bullet, they unconsciously change their minds and jerk their hands away, so that the bullet lands in the room instead of in them.

Similarly, those who slit their wrists often first make "hesitation marks" or parallel slashes with a razor or knife. Rarely do suicides make a deep fatal incision the first time, but rather they seem to test their method, or perhaps the strength of their conviction to die. (Right-handed people usually slash from left to right and the hesitation marks are found on the left; the reverse is generally true for left-handed people.) Such slash marks are often found even when people kill themselves by other means, for many shootings or overdoses of barbiturates are reverted to after an attempted slashing. The suicide switches to another method on seeing that slashing himself is too bloody, too painful, or too slow a death. Some switch methods, however, because the first did not work. People who slash their throats usually throw their heads back, and wrist-slashers have a tendency to flick their wrists outward; both groups thereby protect the very arteries that they were trying to reach.

If no suicide weapon is found, it is usually an indication of homicide—but not always. A man once returned home and hours later died from a bullet wound in his head. No gun or bullet was found, and the medical detectives examining his wound concluded that he must have shot himself earlier and survived after the bullet passed through his brain and out the top of his head. The police checked the hotel he had visited that afternoon and there found the missing bullet and gun.

Suicides are generally stationary, however, as they wait to die, whereas a murder victim often tries to reach the telephone or door for help. Therefore the place in which the body is found, in relation to where he was injured (as established by bloodstains), helps to determine suicide or homicide. Where a person is found is also important. "Jumpers," for example, can only jump as far out in the air as they could have jumped on the ground. Jumpers do not always realize this, and think that, like Superman, they can leap through the air and bypass the net below. Many murderers do not realize this either and have been caught only because they threw the body farther out a window than he could possibly have jumped himself.

Incidentally, another way to determine whether a person jumped or fell from a height, according to Dr. M. Dorothea Kerr, a medical investigator in Manhattan, is by the evidence found underneath his fingernails. A few years ago Dr. Kerr was getting a number of cases of Bowery bums who had supposedly jumped from windows. She noticed that foreign substances were often found under their fingernails. These scrapings showed that they had tried to grab on to something as they were falling, and she realized that this would probably not be true of suicides, who would have chosen to jump down and so would have no reason to stop themselves. She reported this to the police, who soon found a ring of murderers who were finding these derelicts, insuring them, tossing them out of windows, and collecting on their policies.

The location of the body itself suggests suicide if the person dies in front of a mirror, for suicides often watch themselves die—probably more out of nervousness than vanity. The location of the fatal wounds on the body is also significant, for homicides tend to aim haphazardly whereas bullets through the heart, in the center of the forehead, or right into the mouth usually indicate suicide. But there have been gory exceptions, such as the time a young girl played that old childhood game with her boyfriend and told him to "close your eyes and open your mouth." Then she calmly shot him in the mouth.

When a person is shot through the temple, which side the gun is aimed from is not important. Amateur detectives erroneously assume that right-handed people do not use their left hands to shoot themselves (or vice versa). It happens. When a right-handed person shoots himself through the left temple, however, the gun must be held close to the head, because, obviously, a person can only stab or shoot himself where he can reach. Exceptions occur when people devise contraptions to act as levers, but usually these devices are found later. Problems have arisen when bullets were shot from more than an arm's length away—by people who triggered the gun with their toes!

The manner in which people kill themselves varies according to sex. Women tend to favor sleeping pills, while men usually choose brave methods such as guns. There is also a tendency for people to imitate the method of suicide that has received recent publicity, and this is especially true in self-immolations or any forms of suicide that are bizarre.

As for the manner of death, electrocution is almost never a method of suicide. It is usually an accident or homicide (especially when the wires are strung around the dead man's genitals). One man connected the bathroom soap dish to the electric outlet in his bedroom, and while his wife was in the bathroom would turn on the bedroom switch. The voltage was not sufficient to kill her, and after a few electrifying experiences, she innocently called in an electrician, who discovered the ruse.

"Autocide" creates another problem for the medical detectives because it is generally believed that car crashes are never consciously suicidal, and this naiveté is reflected in the fact that automobiles are not even listed in the suicide statistics as instruments of self-destruction. Evidence shows, however, that many auto accidents have indeed been deliberate. Dr. John Edland, chief medical examiner of Monroe County, New York, studied many of these questionable crashes and found that a large number of the drivers had threatened or attempted suicide or had undergone severe personal crises at the time that they got into their car. Yet there is such a reluctance to accept driving as a method of suicide that in one crash in which a suicide motive existed, a note was found, and the circumstances indicated clear intent, the death certificate nonetheless listed the death as "accidental." The coroner who signed the death certificate insisted that "the man obviously had an accident while he was trying to kill himself."

The families and friends of the deceased sometimes play medical detective by deciding that suicide could not have been the cause of death; their kin, they say, was too vain or cowardly to choose that method. Ernest Hemingway's widow, for example, was convinced that her husband would not have shot off the top of his head, leaving only his mouth, chin, and part of his cheeks, because, she said, he would never have allowed himself to be found in that condition. But no matter how algophobic the person is while living, he is often impervious to pain when preparing to die. Some "cowards" have practically decapitated themselves, driven nails into their skulls, used homemade guillotines, crucified themselves, or fastened explosives to their bodies and celebrated the Fourth of July. One woman cut off both her feet plus one hand, and then used her remaining hand to stab herself until she expired. In one especially gruesome incident, a mentally disturbed forty-six-year-old man threw himself under a moving train and cut his body almost in half. One hundred and five pounds of his legs, hips, and pelvis were in one place, and the remaining seventy-five pounds were elsewhere, alive, and in no pain, since the blood vessels had been crushed shut by the pressure. He helped his rescuers, talked with them, even sang, before dying five and a half hours later from shock while undergoing surgery.

Although the manner of death can be meaningless, the manner in which the person is dressed is important in determining suicide. Suicides often open their collars before slashing their throats, or unbutton their shirts before shooting themselves in the chest. Murderers rarely remove or rearrange their victim's clothes, unless rape is involved, in which case the injuries are clearly not self-inflicted. More important is whether the deceased is wearing any clothes at all. Women almost never let themselves be found naked, even after death. Their modesty is reflected in the fact that they rarely disfigure themselves either, so that a woman found naked or grossly disfigured probably did not commit suicide. In fact, female feelings about this run so strong that women who have committed suicide by strangulation in a bathtub are sometimes found fully dressed in the water.

While all of the above are *clues*, there is only one conclusive indication of suicide. If a dead person is found clenching the weapon *tightly*, there is no doubt that he committed suicide. At the moment of death, especially when it occurs under emotional circumstances, a violent muscular reaction can occur, called a cadaveric spasm. This reaction causes the person to grip anything he was holding at the time of his death.

Murderers are usually unaware of this spasm and

often place a gun or knife in the dead person's hand to make it look as if he killed himself. But a cadaveric spasm grip cannot be simulated. As Dr. John Devlin says, when the medical detectives come across a loosely held gun, murder is a possibility, because the gun often either falls out of a suicide's hand or is gripped by this spasm. On the other hand, if they find a tightly gripped murder weapon they *know* the person killed himself.

One medically knowledgeable murderer tried to outwit the medical detectives by tying the victim's hand to the gun after killing him and then waiting for rigor mortis to stiffen his hold, in order to simulate a cadaveric spasm. The medical detectives later found a gun held by a flabby grip, and—more incriminating—physical evidence that something had been tied to the dead man's hand after death.

Cadaveric spasms have proved important in determining homicides as well, for victims sometimes pull hairs and buttons off their assailants as they are being murdered. The spasm provides the clue to track down the murderer.

A cadaveric spasm also can show whether a person was drowned or thrown into water after death. It is proverbial that a drowning man will grasp at any straw, and while there are no straws underwater, there may be weeds or wood. A drowning man will grab at those, and if he experiences cadaveric spasm at death (as happened to one of the brides in the bath) the evidence may be found in the hand to prove that the person was alive when he entered the water.

Without the cadaveric spasm, however, there is no absolute rule that determines a death by suicide as opposed to murder. Sometimes death is a little bit of both, as happened in the following case, which was officially classified as a suicide. A woman took sleeping pills and then pinned a note to her blouse stating, "If you love me, wake me up." Her husband came home at eleven o'clock that night, read the note, crumpled it up, threw it in the wastebasket, and went off to spend the night at a bar. When he returned home the next morning she was dead. It is not surprising that for a while the district attorney debated bringing homicide charges against the husband.

Usually homicides and suicides are more easily distinguishable than that, but when the medical detectives have to decide whether death is suicidal rather than natural or accidental, the clues become thinner and more nebulous than they are for homicide. For example, Keith Simpson, an English medical detective, related the story of an old man who tried to climb up on a high table upon which he had prepared a suicidal gas bed. When he was found dead, the gas had not been turned on yet. His death resulted from a heart attack caused by the physical exertion of trying to get up on the table.

Another time, a man shot himself through the mouth, but it was discovered during the autopsy that the real cause of death was a ruptured aorta. This is a very painful death, and there were indications that the man had tried to get relief in a manner other than suicide. Failing that, he had shot himself to end his misery. The actual cause of death, however, was a natural ailment, and this comforted his family, which could not understand why he would want to kill himself.

Many cases are borderline, and whether cause of death ultimately is registered as an accident, natural death as above, or a suicide depends on the preference of the medical detective. Even if the information available to them were the same throughout the country (which it is not because police work differs) their interpretations would differ. Some categorize an overdose of barbiturates as an accident while others call it suicide.

The decision of suicide may also reflect the way that the death is reported. The fact that one state or country has more suicides than another actually may not reflect on the people who live there, or the way the environment impinges upon them, so much as how suicide is reported. California, for example, has the highest suicide rate in the country, and while there has been speculation that it has something to do with the type of people who choose to live there, or the effect of the area upon them, it should not be overlooked that California keeps very accurate statistical records. In California it is rare to attribute a suicide to "accidental" or "natural" causes for the sake of the family.

It has also been noted that countries which do much for the individual, such as Sweden, have extremely high suicide rates. (Contrary to popular opinion, however, Sweden does not have the highest suicide rate. Hungary is first. Sweden ranks fifth.) But these places may also do more for the individual after he dies. In Russia, for example, everyone who dies in a hospital is autopsied—a fact which may include a more probing analysis into the cause of death, and more honest reporting, than in other countries.

It is also often hard to distinguish suicides from accidents because some people who appear to be contemplating or attempting suicide end by dying accidentally. For example, people who have turned on the gas to die have lit a cigarette (perhaps while considering their decision) and accidentally died from the subsequent explosion. One determined suicide scaled a tree with a bottle of poison, a razor blade, and a rope. As he climbed up the tree, he drank the poison. After he tied the noose he slashed his wrists, and then he hung himself from the noose. But the poison was not strong enough to kill him, the slashes were not deep enough, and the noose broke from the weight of his body. He died accidentally from the fall from the tree.

While he obviously planned to die—albeit not in the manner in which it ultimately occurred—some of the most difficult decisions for the medical detectives arise when a person is known to have reason to kill himself, may have threatened to do so, and is then found dead under conditions which could be accidental. This sometimes happens with an unmarried pregnant woman whose death may result either accidentally from trying to abort her baby, or deliberately in suicide. The same problems are occasionally encountered with unrequited love, as happened in one weird case, where a young boy, rejected by a girl, threatened suicide. The medical detectives later decided that he had probably not been serious but had planned merely to get sick enough to gain her pity so she would return to him. To accomplish this, he took an icy bath in the middle of winter, and then stood naked and wet in front of the kitchen window so that he would catch a cold. When he felt no signs of a cold coming on, he tried to facilitate matters by leaning out of the window to expose more of his body to the inclement weather. His feet were wet from the bath, the kitchen floor was slippery, and he accidentally fell five floors to his death.

Finally, some people who have wanted to die but lacked the courage to commit suicide have compromised by performing a type of semi-suicide so that their life becomes a living death. This was once common in China, where "suicide" was not meant to end life but rather to get back at the person who spoiled it. The victim was always present to enjoy his revenge. In the 1930s in China, for example, it was common for a rejected spouse to drink less than a lethal dose of lye, which can lead to permanent crippling. A woman about to lose her husband to another woman might do that so that her disfigurement would be a constant punishing reminder to the errant husband of his role in its causation.

It should be obvious by now that deciding whether death is suicidal is not clear-cut, that suicide is often relative, and that the classification may reflect primarily the personal biases of the medical detectives. Dr. Robert Litman, chief psychiatrist at the Suicide Prevention Center in Los Angeles, suggests that rather than just labeling all self-inflicted deaths as suicide, we should divide them into degrees, like homicide. First-degree suicide would be deliberate, second-degree impulsive, and third-degree would encompass that nebulous category currently classified as suicide, but which can as readily be accidental—for example, the woman who takes an overdose of sleeping pills expecting her husband to save her: if he is delayed, she dies.

Litman has also suggested that one category of suicide should include what is now classified as accidental or natural death, that is, reckless driving, chronic alcoholism, chain smoking, or drug overdose. The problem is that this would apply to so many people that we would have to accept the depressing (although probably true) notion that every day we all commit suicide little by little.

To review the first case before explaining whether it was suicide or homicide: remember that both shots left the young corporal disfigured; the instantaneously fatal head wound, which caused very little bleeding, was fired twelve to eighteen inches away from her left eye and came out above her right ear, and when she was found her left hand lay loosely over the left breast wound, which had bled extensively.

It would have made things easy for the medical detective had she been found clutching her breast in a cadaveric spasm, for then he would have concluded this was suicide. But her hand was loose. He therefore had to weigh all other evidence too. He knew that the girl's lover had told the truth when he said the first shot was in the breast, and that the second in the head, because the breast wound had bled a lot, while the head wound had not, and furthermore, as stated, death had to have been instantaneous from the second shot.

From there on, the lover was in trouble with his story. First of all, women do not usually choose to shoot themselves and are even less apt to disfigure themselves, although it should be clear from this chapter that there are exceptions to every rule (except cadaveric spasm) and no one could arrive at a conclusion based on that evidence alone.

The important thing, however, was the angle of the fatal bullet. This showed which hand she would have had to have used to pull the trigger. It is easier to understand this if you turn your index finger into an imaginary gun, and bring your right hand over to your left eye at such an angle that the bullet could come out above your right ear, as happened in this case. It is an extremely awkward angle. And if you keep that same position and pull your hand twelve to eighteen inches away (which was the distance of the gun in this case) it is obviously almost impossible.

The alternative was that the girl had used her left

hand for the fatal shot in the head, but that could not have been, for her left hand was clutching the first wound on her breast. The only other possibility, that she had shot herself in the left temple with her left hand, dropped the gun, and grabbed the first wound with the same hand was impossible since death from the second head wound was instantaneous.

If she could not have used her right hand, therefore (because of the angle), or her left hand (because it was on her breast), her lover's hand must have fired the gun. The jury agreed with the medical detective and the officer was given life imprisonment.

9

Paternity Suits

A man was living with a woman who had six children, and he married her when she told him that he was the father of her seventh child. Later, certain things came to light that made him wonder if the child was really his. He ordered blood tests in hopes of finding grounds for the annulment of their marriage. She had type O, he had type B, and the child was type AB. Could the child have been theirs?

Although the who-done-it in criminology traditionally means who committed the crime, in the field of paternity, which also is handled by the medical detectives, the who-done-it means who fathered the child. It is a question that has bothered society since time immemorial. And it is not just a theoretical problem, for a man convicted of a paternity charge can be ordered to pay anywhere from $100 to $1,200 a year over a sixteen- to twenty-one-year period for support of the child, not to mention the cost to his reputation in business and social circles.

In ancient China problems of paternity were solved simply, if unscientifically, by having the man and the child in question cut their fingers over a bowl. If the blood mixed smoothly, they were believed to be related; if not, the child was said not to be his. The ancient Carthaginians had another way of solving the problem. They would bring the baby at two months of age before a special committee that would decide whether it bore any resemblance to the purported father. If the baby failed the test, they had an equally simple solution to the problem: it was destroyed.

In "modern" America the issue is often just as unscientifically decided, despite the fact that the medical detectives have certain tests at their disposal which if properly performed are infallible.

Briefly, some red blood cells have certain agglutinins labeled A and B; if the cells have both, they are called type AB; if they have neither, they are called type O. A blood factor cannot appear in the blood of a child unless it is present in the blood of either the mother or father, and no factor in the child's blood can be foreign to the blood of both of his parents. Thus, two type B parents cannot have a type A child; two type O parents can give birth only to another type O, and so on. (In addition, a number of subgroups, such as MN, Rh-Hr or Kell, subdivide the population further.)

Parenthetically, it should be mentioned that it is now sometimes possible scientifically to determine paternity even before a child is born. According to *Newsweek*, a woman in Sweden wanted to make certain that her future child was the son of her husband (who was black) and not of her lover (who was white), for if the latter were true she wanted an abortion. The doctors removed a small quantity of amniotic fluid, analyzed the chromosomes of the fetal cells, and saw that they contained characteristics of her husband. They were apparently right, for five months later she gave birth to a black child.

Rather than relying on these tests, however, some courts of law choose superstition over science. The most famous travesty occurred when Joan Berry claimed that Charles Chaplin was the father of her child. Joan Berry had type O. Chaplin had type A. The child had type B and, given his type O mother, could have been sired only by a type AB or type B father. Furthermore, Chaplin insisted that he had stopped seeing her thirteen months before she gave birth, but she asked the jury to believe the unlikely story that she had broken into his house four months after they broke up, walked into the bedroom, threatened him with a gun, that they stopped arguing long enough to make love, after which she took the gun out and again threatened him. This jury did believe it and Chaplin was ruled to be the father.

Several states still permit superficial resemblance to be counted as evidence in a paternity trial, and this was also true during the Chaplin case when the child was held up in court next to him so the jury could determine whether they looked alike. Other, more enlightened states, while not permitting anything about resemblance actually to be articulated, allow the putative parent to bring the baby into the courtroom. Sometimes it is not necessary to discuss resemblance at all, as happened, for example, when a black man brought an infant into the courtroom and claimed that an Italian was the real father. The picture of the white baby on his lap said more than a thousand words to the jury.

Not only do some courts ignore scientific evidence, they make it as difficult as possible for the defendant to present it. The man accused of being the father is generally the one who must pay for the blood tests to prove his innocence, a fact which obviously often acts as a deterrent to ordering them. Many innocent men choose to quit rather than fight, and even if they do choose the latter course, only a few states force a jury to accept the scientific blood evidence. Sometimes the jury may discount general medical evidence as well. In one case in which it could be proved that the putative father had not seen the mother for one year before the birth of her child, he was adjudged to be the father anyway. Another time a doctor once testified in court that the defendant had too low a sperm count to father any child, but the jury ruled that he should pay for the support of the child on the ground that "it only takes one sperm to impregnate anyway."

Even where blood tests are used and accepted, a problem arises, because no blood test can prove that a man is definitely the father of the child; it can only prove, at times, that he is *not.* The reason it is impossible to determine with absolute certainty that a particular man fathered a baby is that the number of blood groups is limited. As a result, many people belong to the same group so that more than one man could be the father of any child. Thus an innocent man with a normal blood constellation has as good a chance of proving by blood type that a child is not his as he has by flipping a coin. Sidney Schatkin, an attorney who has handled more than 1,100 paternity cases, explains that as a result, "If one hundred women in America arbitrarily chose one hundred men in China and insisted that they were the fathers of their babies, only about fifty of the men could definitely prove otherwise with blood tests."

For many years the Scandinavians had a system which encouraged women to disclose the paternity of their child. A woman had only to state which men *could have been* the father and *all* of them would have to pay the full (small) amount for support. The mother would get one portion to help bring up her child, and the rest went to children whose fathers could not be found or could not afford to pay. (This policy was stopped in the mid 1960s for fear that it might have a traumatic effect on the child to discover that many men could have been the father.)

But in America, many women have found that it literally pays to lie, for often they get away with it. More than one woman has insisted that only two men could have fathered their babies and when both were tested, neither turned out to be the one. One young girl was adamant that only the accused could have fathered her child, insisting that she had never slept with another man. When the blood tests exonerated him, she became so distraught that her attorney was almost ready to believe in immaculate conception. He was rudely awakened when, having presented his bill, she offered to take the sum out with him in trade!

Although some women make preposterous claims about who impregnated them, others tell even more outlandish tales about how they got in that condition—even though there is only one known way to get there. One girl admitted in court that she had not had intercourse with the alleged father; indeed, she was not even certain if he had ejaculated. While medical literature contains cases of impregnation without completion of copulation, and while certain physical anomalies have enabled women to get pregnant through rectal or urethral intercourse, in this case, the plaintiff admitted that all the defendant had done was to "fool around with his fingers." But since she swore on a Bible that she had never had intercourse with any man in her life, the jury decided that her pregnancy must indeed have occurred in this unique manner and the man was ordered to support her child.

In an even more ridiculous situation, a woman swore that she had been impregnated on a public street one night while she and her lover were both standing at a corner. While this might be possible if not quite proper, she added that no penetration had occurred. What happened, she claimed, was that she had her period and was wearing a sanitary napkin which her lover ejaculated upon, causing her to become pregnant.

The judge did not believe it either.

The medical detectives or serologists who work on paternity cases are the same ones who type the blood found on suspected murderers to see if it matches the victim's; type the blood found on a victim to see if it might have come from a suspected assailant; or type semen in a rape case. Some of their work is in another area—establishing whether "twins" are related.

For example, there have been cases in which the blood types proved that a man was not the father of onc twin, but it could not establish that he was not the father of the other. This usually occurs because the child's blood type is not strong enough to allow the father to be "excluded," as it is called. However, the occurrence brings up another interesting and little-known phenomenon called "superfecundation." This happens when a female has intercourse with two different males at close intervals. Two eggs are released, and two children are born, each by a different father. Superfecundation is known to occur among animals, but in humans it is extremely rare (some doctors believe an impossibility), despite certain cases reported in the early medical literature. And since it occurs rarely (if at all), when this question of twins with different fathers has come to court in contemporary times, the court has always recognized the possibility of superfecundation and always ruled against it, saying that neither twin belonged to the putative father. Thus both children are stamped illegitimate, despite the minute possibility that through this strange phenomenon at least one of them could be the progeny of the alleged father.

One interesting case involving blood typing of twins had its beginnings in Switzerland and was ultimately solved here in America. A Swiss couple, both identical twins themselves, gave birth to twins. When the boys were about five years old, the parents spent an evening with a couple whom they had never met before. During the evening, this new couple introduced their child to them, and to their astonishment he looked exactly like one of their twins. The first couple went home and tried to forget the coincidence, but they were so disturbed by the strength of the resemblance that they returned to see this couple the next day to discuss the situation with them further. It was then that they discovered that this child who looked exactly like one of their boys had been born on the same day as their sons. And at the same hospital.

The parents visited the head of the hospital, who assured them that there was no way the boys possibly could have been mixed up and given to the wrong parents. But they were not so sure. The two couples decided to have blood tests done on their children, but the facilities were limited in Switzerland. Only a few broad tests could be done and these proved inconclusive. The Swiss doctor suggested that they contact Dr. Alexander Wiener, co-discoverer of the Rh factor, and director of the serological and bacteriological laboratories at the Office of the Chief Medical Examiner in New York City, perhaps the most famous medical detective in the world in the field of serology.

Because of the nature of blood tests, Dr. Wiener could not state for sure who was related to whom, for the same reason that no serologist can state with certainty that one baby is definitely the child of a certain man. But as in paternity cases, he could show who was *not* related. With blood tests, then, he proved that one of the "twins" of the first couple could not be their child, that the boy of the other family could not be theirs, and that the two "twins" who had been brought up together could not be brothers. That was certainly sufficient. Incredibly enough, the parents switched children, and the single child went off to live as a twin and one of the "twins" went with the first family. Much later, when the boys were asked how they liked the change, each said that he liked his new family better than the earlier one, and one of the boys gave his reason. "My new family has a bigger car," he boasted.

The woman in the first case had type O blood, the father had type B, and the child had type AB. The man and woman could not, therefore, have produced the child, for someone had to give it the type A factor. But the strange element in this case (Dr. Wiener's) was that the woman was not the mother either. It turned out that the mother had had a hysterectomy after her sixth child, and had got the child from an orphanage in order to hook her lover into marriage. He got the annulment he wanted.

10

Rape

An eight-year-old girl was found strangled and stuffed in a sack in a small apartment house in Scotland, and her badly damaged sexual organs suggested a motive to the crime. The famous English pathologist Sir Sydney Smith, the medical detective who performed the autopsy, saw that this did not appear to be a case of someone trying to cover up murder by rape, for the girl clearly had been raped first and murdered shortly after. He also noticed that the girl had an enlarged thymus, and he wondered if it may have played some role in the murder, since people who have this condition sometimes go into a coma from the slightest shock.

The assailant was believed to have been someone who lived in her apartment building, because the sack she was found in was dry although it had been raining outside. The police questioned all the men who lived there and soon narrowed the suspects to one man. He and his wife did not get along with the child and they were the only people in the building who had not joined in the search for her when she first disappeared. But this man, like all of the others in the building, had an excellent alibi. What happened and who done it?

Rape, which derives from the Latin verb "to seize," requires three elements which cannot be always corroborated by physical evidence: carnal or sexual knowledge, force, and lack of consent. While it would seem that the first, carnal knowledge, would leave the most obvious sign in the form of semen, rape legally does not require ejaculation, or even penetration. It is considered a fait accompli if a man enters only the vulva or outer lips of the vagina, and as a result there may not be physical evidence to confirm it.

It is often hard to prove physical force, and as a result, the victim's word of whether rape occurred is sometimes the sole determinant—and rarely believed. Cervantes tells in *Don Quixote* of a buxom woman who went to court to accuse a man of rape. The woman claimed that she had met the man in a deserted place, and while she screamed and fought with all of her maidenly might, he had easily forced the issue. The man admitted that carnal knowledge had indeed occurred, but he insisted that the only force he utilized was to fight off the overanxious female. The governor and judge of the Province, Sancho Panza, ruled in favor of the woman and ordered the defendant to turn over all the money in his pockets as recompense. Which he did. But as they were leaving the courtroom, Sancho called the man back and told him he could have his money back *if* he could take it away from the woman. The two struggled, but the woman fought so hard that he could not get near either her or the purse. Whereat the judge ordered the woman to return the man's money, explaining, with the sagaciousness of Solomon, that had she fought as hard to hold onto her virtue as she did for her money, he could never have forced her to intercourse.

Lack of consent usually accompanies force or the threat of force and it, too, can be difficult to corroborate, especially since *legally* the woman does not have to withhold her consent throughout the entire act. In actual fact, indication of consent or pleasure at any time *is* held against her, and many a rape case has been thrown out of court when it came out that the girl kissed the man goodnight afterward.

A woman is expected to indicate her reluctance clearly. There is the perhaps apocryphal story of the young girl who insisted in a courtroom that she had been raped by the defendant, although she said she had made it verbally clear to the man that she was not consenting to his activities.

"Why didn't you shout for help?" the man's lawyer wanted to know.

"I didn't want to wake up my mother, who was sleeping in the next room," she answered.

Lack of consent does not always accompany force, as, for example, when the woman was drunk and asleep at the time and incapable of protest.

It is generally accepted that a woman cannot be raped in her sleep without waking up, and this problem arose in England in the nineteenth century when a woman went to sleep around midnight. At two A.M., while she was in that hypnogogic state between waking and sleeping, she became aware that she was having intercourse and assumed that the man was her husband. As she woke up completely from the act, the man lying in bed with her pushed her nightgown over her head and ran away. It was only as she pushed her gown back down that she glimpsed the fleeing man and saw that he was a stranger. The man was caught eventually and brought to trial. The judge ruled the woman was raped because her consent had been obtained by fraudulent means.

Rape by fraud still occasionally comes up in court, as in the case of a singing teacher who convinced a student that intercourse would improve her voice—it was considered rape. Today, however, the law states that a woman is not raped if she consents under fraudulent conditions. If she thinks her marriage is legal when it is not, or if a doctor falsely represents sexual intercourse as part of her medical treatment and she consents, she has not been raped. But if she was deceived about the situation—if the doctor tells her he is just giving her a typical gynecological examination and he substitutes his penis for his speculum—it is rape.

If a woman claims she was raped, or if the medical detective is trying to establish whether a dead woman was raped, he will search for signs of carnal knowledge, force, and lack of consent, even though physical proof is difficult to establish. The first procedure is to look for spermatazoa—actually one spermatazoon will suffice. The second is to ascertain that it is of human and not animal origin.

The third step is to search for blood and bodily injuries consistent with force and lack of consent. Where they look for these injuries depends upon the age of the victim. Older women who are used to sex, especially those who have borne children, are not likely to suffer damage to their sexual organs by rape, although they may have bruises elsewhere on their body (especially on their shoulder blades and buttocks if they were pinned down). However, if two or more men rape a woman, she is less likely to have bruises than if just one does it for at least one of the men usually holds her down and prevents her from struggling or fighting. In children, however, the sex organs are generally torn, and, incidentally, only among young children is the rape itself the sole cause of death.

The clothes worn by attacker and victim also can provide clues as to whether or not rape occurred. They may have semen on them, pubic hair, and rips and tears which help support the woman's claim of a struggle. Sometimes it tells the opposite story. Once, a well-developed eleven-year-old girl complained to her parents that she had been molested by a fourteen-year-old after he invited her to his home to look at his comic books. She said he had pulled down her underpants, tried to penetrate her, and that "it hurt." She said this all occurred when she went over there as the siren of the local mill blew seven o'clock. The boy's father, however, was employed by that nearby mill, and claimed that when he had come home two to four minutes after the whistle blew, the girl was not in his house.

The girl had been dressed in a complicated outfit with underclothes so much too long for her that her mother had shortened them with a safety pin. If the neighbor's boy had pulled them off, as she said, they would have been ripped at the safety pin. They had not. If, on the other hand, he had unpinned and removed what was practically a chastity belt, it would have taken a minimum of one and a half minutes, as estimated on a mannikin. The conclusion was that it was impossible for the girl to have gone to the boy's house, been undressed, assaulted, and returned home in four minutes, a conclusion strengthened when it was learned later that the girl had been punished at school for raising her skirt to the boys.

Carnal knowledge can sometimes be corroborated by

venereal disease, and in one situation this had a curious twist. Two young girls accused a sailor of rape, and their claim seemed to be supported when a doctor testified in court that both girls had contracted gonorrhea. But later in the trial, another doctor testified that the sailor did not have the disease, and it later developed that these two Lolitas were so promiscuous that the "rapist" could consider himself lucky to have caught nothing from them.

All these things, then, provide confirmation of rape: semen, VD, bruises, blood, pubic hair, or clothes. In addition, some men feel they can find subtle evidence in the victim's behavior. One police surgeon claims that whenever he tells a woman who claims to have been raped to lie down on the examination table so he can look for physical evidence of rape, the way she spreads her legs and the position that she takes will tell the entire story.

Although most claims of rape are probably true, the medical literature tends to report more of the opposite instances. Occasionally the doctors themselves are the victims, and dentists and physicians are sometimes accused by their patients of raping them after anaesthetizing them. This is because the drugs may cause erotic hallucinations which lead the patient to believe that more than imagination was at play. And cases have been reported in which the person who makes the claim really was sexually used—but not by a man. A few young girls have turned out to be victimized or used by their own mothers, some of whom make Medea look like the Madonna. A ten-year-old girl with unnatural-looking sex organs eventually admitted to the doctor that it was not a man, but her mother who had systematically dilated her vagina with her fingers and finally inserted a long stone into her so that she would be "prepared to have intercourse with men." Another mother put her twelve-year-old daughter into her husband's bed and encouraged the two to have intercourse, because she said she "couldn't be bothered" with it herself.

One psychotic mother hysterically insisted that her eleven-year-old daughter had been raped by a local shopkeeper, a highly respected member of the community. The child was found to have gonorrhea, which seemed to corroborate the mother's accusation. But it came out during the court trial that the mother had tried to extort money from this shopkeeper, and failing to collect, turned her daughter over to her own lover, who was as depraved as she was. He raped her in order to provide the medical evidence to support the mother's charges. It was the lover, not the shopkeeper, who had VD.

On the other hand, sometimes it's the children who are in need of psychiatric help. A child was once brought to the police station after making charges of rape against her father. He was brought in with her—under arrest. Physical examination of the child not only indicated that she was a virgin, but that she had an imperforate hymen which would have to be operated on before she could have intercourse.

Another time, in St. Louis, a ten-year-old girl accused a local garage mechanic of having raped her, and while that may or may not have been true on that occasion, it was discovered that she had voluntarily visited him eleven times for sexual purposes before complaining to the police about his forcible advances.

In one case, the medical detectives thought they had found evidence of rape, but actual events turned out to have little to do with sex. A woman was found dead in a ditch in England, and when the medical detectives saw the severe damage to her genitals, they immediately concluded that she had been the victim of a vicious rape. But when they examined these vulval injuries further, they realized that something larger and heavier than a human organ had entered her. The police later found a young boy who admitted that he had been speeding on his bicycle on the night in question when he suddenly rode over a woman who was facing him as she squatted by the side of the road to urinate. The handlebars had struck her in the face and neck and the front wheel of his bike had driven into her vagina. He left her there in the road, where she soon died from loss of blood. The boy was convicted of manslaughter—not rape.

The medical detectives sometimes examine deceased *males* to determine if they were victims of sodomous acts, because homosexuality often plays a role in murder or suicide. This is partly due to society's general lack of tolerance for the homosexual, which can cause them to experience guilt, disgrace, and blackmail, and also the promiscuity of many homosexuals, since that can lead to suspicion, jealousy, and ultimately murder. (In murder trials, the law tends to favor the heterosexual, as in the case of one father who beat a homosexual to death with his bare hands when he found him having oral intercourse with his nine-year-old son. He was acquitted under justifiable homicide.) Hustlers who prey on homosexuals can be especially dangerous, for if the victim resists, they may kill him. The hustler usually goes free, invariably pleading that he defended himself from the advances of a homosexual.

If a man was raped, there may be physical damage to his anus, if it was his first homosexual act, if there was a gross disparity in the size of parts (as when a grown man rapes a child), or if considerable violence was used. But the medical detectives can also investigate allegations of rape by checking to see if the victim was accustomed to homosexuality (determined by healed scars in the anal region, a funnel-shaped orifice, or an unduly wide canal); by searching for semen or pubic hair in or on the victim, and by examining the alleged assailant for semen, pubic hair, fecal material, or anal secretions on his sexual organs or clothes—especially his underclothes.

There have been almost no cases in medical history of women committing a sex "crime" against a man. For example, if a man is caught watching a woman undress, he may find himself in jail as a Peeping Tom. But if a woman is caught watching a man take off his clothes, *he* may be arrested for exhibitionism. Still, a couple of cases have brought up the old question of whether it is possible for a woman to rape a man.

In America, the law states that rape cannot be committed directly by a woman, but she can be convicted of a statutory offense of having carnal knowledge of and sexual intercourse with an infant. In France, however, an eighteen-year-old girl was tried for the rape of two boys, one eleven and the other thirteen. The boys claimed that she enticed them into the fields, and then forced them to have intercourse with her, although exactly how she accomplished this feat is not known. *Why* she did, however, was revealed at her trial, for it seems that she suffered from a physiologically abnormal contraction of the vaginal musculature, which made it impossible for her to have intercourse with an adult male. Whether or not she really forced the issue, or simply let nature take its course, is subject to question, but the boys seemed to be telling the truth that some sex had occurred, because surprisingly she had syphilis, and after she had finished with the boys, so did they. She was convicted of rape and sentenced, incredibly enough, to fifteen years hard labor.

It will be remembered that the medical detective in the opening case had determined that the dead girl had an enlarged thymus, that she had been raped before she died, that damage to her genitals was extensive, as would be expected in a child her age, and that she was disliked by a couple in the building. The husband, however, had an undisputed alibi for the time that she died. From forensic knowledge and clues the medical detective reconstructed the crime as follows:

The wife of the suspect also hated the child, and perhaps some kind of altercation had transpired that day which led to the woman's shaking or slapping her. Because of the girl's enlarged thymus, she suddenly collapsed from this slight provocation and the wife then thought that she had killed her. She decided to divert suspicion from herself and "raped" the girl by inserting some object (either a poker or a broom handle) into her so it would look like a man had done the deed. The excruciating pain caused the girl to suddenly regain consciousness, since someone heard a child scream at that time. The mother, realizing her mistake, and knowing that she could never explain to the child or her parents what she had been doing and why, then panicked and quickly strangled the child.

She was sentenced to ten years in jail.

11

Drugs

Dr. J. M. Lehotay, acting chief medical examiner of Erie County, New York, is different from most medical detectives. For one thing, she is a woman. Second—and this could well be related to the first—Dr. Lehotay does not always share the detached demeanor of some of her male colleagues. She sometimes becomes emotionally involved in her cases. Her round, blue eyes occasionally seem to fight back tears as she talks about her work, and she is not embarrassed to admit that some of these deaths "upset" her, make her "unable to sleep," and even cause her to "almost cry."

While such an attitude might be greeted with guffaws by some male medical detectives, no one who knows her laughs. Instead, most people develop a protective attitude toward her, and some of her male colleagues have even gotten involved with *her* case. Dr. Lehotay's special problem is sexual discrimination in a traditionally male occupation. At the current time, Dr. Judith Lehotay is the *acting* chief medical examiner of Erie County, but she has not been appointed chief medical examiner. And the position is available—but so far not for a woman.

Dr. Lehotay is not the only female medical detective who is currently facing sexual discrimination. Dr. Clara Raven in Michigan, for example, is battling the same problem. According to Dr. Raven, she was "certified by the Civil Service for the job of chief medical examiner . . . [and] rated first in a promotional examination, but the appointment was never finalized." Today she is *deputy* chief medical examiner and, like Dr. Lehotay, has been interim acting chief—but never the chief. In response to the question of whether there is anything inherent in the job of medical examiner that a man can do better than a woman, Dr. Raven laughs.

"During the Algiers Motel incident (when three people were killed, nine were beaten, and reports of snipers were rampant) all the male doctors were afraid to go out and stayed home for the first few days. *I* was the only doctor with the courage to go out," she chuckles.

On the other hand, Dr. Jane Simon of the New York City Medical Examiner's Office (probably the only medical detective ever to wear hot pants at the scene of a murder) finds her sex an asset, though she does tire of the policemen who take one look at her when she walks onto the scene and exclaim: "*You're* the doctor?" She says that being a female does have its advantages when she is testifying in court. This diminutive thirty-year-old doctor finds that the lawyers on the other side seem afraid to subject her to a grueling cross-examination, and that those who try are stopped by the judges, who have a protective and paternal attitude toward her.

Despite the discrimination, Dr. Lehotay considers herself lucky to have achieved her high position. She is lucky in other ways too, lucky to be alive, for this Hungarian-born doctor almost didn't make it through the 1956 uprising. When the Russians marched into Hungary, she got involved: "How can you stay home and stay out of it when you're a physician and people all around you are dying?" she asks. "So I improvised a hospital and gave first aid to the students who were injured while fighting the Russians. But when we lost, I knew that the Russians were about ready to hang me two times over."

She and her husband escaped from the country quickly with the assistance of the Hungarian border patrol. But as their escape necessitated their being totally silent over a long period of time, they could not chance taking along their ten-month-old son. Having left him behind, they did not come to America right after their escape but instead stayed near Hungary and plotted ways to sneak him out of the country.

While waiting, they heard of a doctor who had devised "sleeping suppositories" that could be inserted into a child to keep him from awakening—exactly the thing for a situation such as this. They provided the doctor with the age and weight of their child and he made up a prescription or a sleeping suppository to be used every three hours. That took care of one problem.

The second was solved when they learned of another refugee who likewise left a son behind. Together they hatched a scheme to get the two boys out.

Both men were aware that there were prices on their heads, and that their former neighbors in Hungary were always on the lookout, waiting for them to return for their children. However since the two men had lived in different neighborhoods, each was unknown to the other's neighbors. So after sneaking back into Hungary, Mr. Lehotay went to the other man's home and kidnapped his son for him, while his friend did the same for Mr. Lehotay. Neither man was recognized, the children remained quiet because of the sleeping prescriptions, and both families were ultimately reunited. Today, the Lehotay's son is sixteen years old and they also have a fourteen-year-old daughter. And despite the discrimination that females face in forensic medicine, the daughter is planning to be a medical examiner one day.

Dr. Lehotay's personal involvement in her work is one of the factors that accounts for her success. One case started when she received a call from the Buffalo police to come along on a "Jane Doe" case, that is, one in which the dead girl's identity is unknown. The call came late at night, and Dr. Lehotay, along with two policemen, had to drive through a very rough neighborhood to reach the victim. It was early in 1970 at a time when policemen were being frequently attacked, and the two policemen grew increasingly nervous as the drive continued. As the streets became more deserted, they began to speculate as to whether there really was a victim, or whether they were being lured into a trap to become the victims themselves.

They continued to talk about the possibility of an ambush, and then, realizing that their statements might frighten a female, they stopped. They did not know that in Hungary, all female medical students are drafted into the army, and Lehotay had been a reserve first lieutenant. When one of the policemen nervously tried to reassure her that she would eventually get home safely, she laughed and told them cheerfully, "If anything happens just throw me a pistol. I may seem soft but I could castrate a fly with a single shot."

When they arrived, there turned out to be no ambush—and there was a body. "She was an absolutely beautiful young black girl," says Dr. Lehotay. "I've never seen anyone so lovely in all my life. Gorgeous long lines. Perfect proportions. I felt so sad to see something so beautiful destroyed. It was like the end of a work of art."

The work of art lay naked on the bed, face down. The first thing Dr. Lehotay suspected was that the girl was a prostitute, which turns out to be the case for many Jane Does. Parenthetically, it might be mentioned that lately the medical detectives are finding that an increased number of John Doe cases are the victims of prostitutes, as these women are becoming increasingly vicious toward their customers. Prostitution, together with homosexuality and gambling, used to be classified as victimless crimes, but this is not always true any more.

Most medical detectives feel that they see more cases today involving victims of prostitutes because many prostitutes are now on drugs. Almost all female drug addicts eventually turn to this obvious source of income to support the spiraling cost of their habit, and like male addicts they may become violent when times are hard. Similarly, rather than drugs leading to prostitution, prostitution sometimes leads to drugs. Many are given cocaine by their pimps, who believe that the drug causes an intensification of sexual desire.

To determine if Jane Doe was a prostitute was not as easy as it would appear. Not every prostitute is as clearly marked as the one in Richmond, Virginia, who had tattooed over one strategic spot: "Pay as you Enter." Dr. Lehotay first looked at the teeth. The girl had a number of cavities. This is often the sign of a drug addict, since heroin use leads to a craving for sweets, and addicts have other things to do than visit dentists. The girl was probably a prostitute if she had to support a habit. (Later, Dr. Lehotay, noting a number of enema bags in the bathroom, checked the girl's rectum. It was funnel-shaped, indicating that she was accustomed to rectal intercourse, and this too gave evidence that she might be a prostitute, for she says that men choose that "route" to avoid venereal disease.)

The next step was to determine when the girl had died. It was March and the weather outside was cold, but the body was still warm. Either the girl had just died or . . . Dr. Lehotay checked the furnace, saw that it was up very high, and realized that body warmth was not a good indicator of death in this case. She checked the eye muscles, flexed the elbows and legs, and saw that rigor mortis was complete, although decomposition had not yet started. She therefore placed the time of the girl's death at about twelve hours earlier.

The final step—establishing what caused the girl to die—was not as simple. Dr. Lehotay first checked to see if the girl had petechial hemorrhages, an indication that she had been asphyxiated. There were none. However, some bloodstained fluid had oozed from the girl's nose and mouth, which could suggest strangulation. On the other hand, it could have come from pulmonary edema, or congestion. This possibility made death from a drug overdose, her first theory, even more likely.

Unfortunately, there was no one telling, for while there was someone else there, he was revealing nothing. When Dr. Lehotay and the policemen had first arrived, a man of about fifty was in the apartment with the girl, waiting for the police. The police soon learned that he had just been released from jail on a drug charge, but the man could not (or would not) shed any light on how the girl had died, or whether her death had anything to do with drugs. He insisted that he did not know the girl who was in his bed, and that he had met her in a neighborhood bar for the first time the night before. He tried to make the nature of her visit to his apartment seem platonic, but with Dr. Lehotay's assertion of prostitution he changed his story and admitted that she was indeed a prostitute. He staunchly denied, however, that she had taken any drugs, or that he had given any to her. He said he did not know when she had died. He had thought she was asleep when he left her that morning. Returning that night and finding her dead, like any good citizen, he had called the police.

But Dr. Lehotay had noticed something odd. Although the neighborhood in which this girl had died was poor, and the apartment house itself (it later proved to be owned by the man) was unimpressive, his own apartment—in which the girl was found—was the ultimate in luxury. As soon as Dr. Lehotay had entered she had been impressed by the gold and marble, the plush carpeting, the fine paintings and expensive items around the apartment. She wondered whether a man would leave a woman whom he did not know—and a prostitute at that—alone in an apartment so sumptuous and filled with so many tempting items. Her feminine intuition said No. If she was right, the man was lying. Either he had never left the apartment during the day, or else he knew that she was dead when he went away in the morning and could safely be left behind. If the first were true, then the man was somehow guilty (even if only by being present when she took drugs); but if he knew that she was already dead when he left his apartment that morning, then his delay in calling the police was even more suspicious. But not much could be done unless Dr. Lehotay could figure out how the girl had died, for only then could she determine whether the man had any part in her death.

The medical detectives' caseload today reflects the alarming increase in hard drugs. (Yet despite the increase in deaths associated with drugs and the resultant publicity, abuse of *alcohol* in this country still leads to more violence than that of drugs. Not only is alcohol often a factor in murder, but half of all people who commit suicide have been drinking as well.) The medical detectives point out that the drugs themselves may not be inherently destructive. The reason that addicts generally die a lot younger than those who are not addicted is because of the way addicts are treated by other addicts, society, or themselves. Another reason is that drugs are illegal and expensive, which forces junkies to perform dangerous acts in order to get enough money to pay for their habits. The drugs themselves may cause death only if a person takes an overdose—and such deaths are rarer than believed, often caused by mixing a drug with central-nervous-system depressants, or from an adverse reaction to the materials with which the drugs are cut. It is believed, for example, that quinine may cause a reaction. Some deaths have been attributed to the fact that an addict sometimes gets drugs that *were not* cut. If the addict is used to heavily diluted material and instead gets a package of strong drugs, he may literally be killed with kindness.

Besides the problems for the medical detectives in the area of the what-done-it, when death is caused by drugs, they sometimes have a problem with how, for it is not uncommon for accidental deaths from drugs to be misinterpreted as suicide or murder. For example, the medical detectives have not yet been able to figure out how to detect the presence of LSD in the body after death, since the average dose can be the equivalent of only 1/30,000th of a regular pill. And yet determining that a person took LSD can mean the difference between classifying a death as accidental or suicidal, for people on LSD sometimes jump out of windows or throw themselves in front of cars with no overtly suicidal intent.

With hard drugs, however, the problem for the medical detectives is usually not in distinguishing accidents versus suicide but rather accidents versus murder. Dr. Michael Baden, deputy medical examiner of Manhattan who has made a specialty of drug cases, explains that in no other area does death so often look homicidal when it is not. He says this is usually because of the addict's friends—often addicts themselves—who may sincerely try to "help" the dying junkie, but more often speed him on his way. Not uncommonly the friends put the dying addict into a cold shower, or they put ice cubes around his testicles, which instead of saving him, as they have erroneously been informed, makes his blood pressure fall even lower than it has already dropped from shock. Dr. Baden says it is also not uncommon for friends to try the home remedy of forcing milk down the dying addict's throat, again in the belief that it will save him, although it may travel down the windpipe and is about as helpful as the ice cubes or cold shower.

Then, after the addict dies, his friends or those around him may attempt to resuscitate him, which can leave suspicious-looking marks or bruises, making the addict look as if he has been in a fight or the victim of violence. Those around him may also try to move him to another location after he dies (so that they won't have any explaining to do to the police) and a body found dumped somewhere is usually immediately assumed to have been murdered. But Dr. Baden complains that just as a medical detective confronted with many such cases gets really adept at spotting a drug death, occasionally an addict is murdered or an addict is found who really *did* commit suicide or died of natural causes. There just is no simple formula here.

Dr. Baden once examined the body of a dead prostitute pocked by the track marks of her drug injections. His first hunch was that she died from drugs. But when he examined her again, he saw that she had faint marks around her neck and arms that looked as if they may have come from a ligature. The only explanation was that she might have been tied up at one time. To add to the mystery, further examination revealed that she had bruises around her mouth. Baden therefore checked for petechial hemorrhages in her eyes, which he found, and he then realized that she had died of asphyxiation rather than drugs. Since she appeared to have been bound, Baden suspected that someone else was probably involved. The police soon tracked down the man who had been with her that night, who turned out to be a doctor of psychology. At first he denied everything—knowing her, being there—but when he was told about the medical evidence, he broke down and told this bizarre tale.

It seems that this man derived sexual pleasure from having prostitutes tie him up and beat him, and then, reversing the process, beating them. He had discovered, the hard way, that once a prostitute had tied him up, she would often grab his money and run, leaving him there without a chance to have any "fun." He usually beat the girls first, therefore, stuffing a gag down their mouths and taping it to prevent them from screaming while he beat them. But on that occasion he stuffed the gag down too deeply and she suffocated. When he saw she was dead, he removed her bonds and the gag and left her, hoping the medical examiner would attribute her death to drugs. Dr. Baden did not.

But such cases are very uncommon. Dr. Lehotay's case was probably the opposite of Dr. Baden's, and far more typical. It looked like a drug death which the man hoped would be attributed to something else. The next day in her office, Dr. Lehotay examined the girl's body for signs of recent drug usage: track marks or signs of recent hemorrhages. She searched for the track marks on the girl's arms—but found no trace of them. As for the hemorrhages, they did not show externally on the girl's dark skin. One can also find hemorrhages by cutting directly into the skin, but as Dr. Lehotay explains: "If you can't see the hemorrhage on the outside, then you don't know where to start. The only way to find it is to keep cutting, and I have too much respect for the bodies to damage them in that way."

Some people might have given up and signed out the cause of death as unknown. But not Dr. Lehotay—she was already too involved in the case. Instead, she consulted the "morgue men," who transport the bodies and prepare them for an autopsy.

"Sure I know that some of the professionals look down on the morgue men," she admits, "but they can really be very helpful. They know all kinds of things that aren't in our medical books. Many of them live in ghetto areas and they sometimes know more about what we're dealing with these days than we do. So I went to the morgue men and told them how I had searched for track marks in her arms and they laughed at my naiveté. They said that addicts were a lot more imaginative than I realized, and they suggested that I look for track marks on the outside of the genitals, in the armpits, in the legs, in the back of the knees and feet, and especially around the ankles where the veins are obvious.

"I took their advice and got a magnifying glass, and sure enough, right there on the inside of her ankle was a very clear mark. I cut into it and found a hemorrhage, a recent one, showing that the injection had to have been administered within twenty-four hours of the time she had died. Since the man in the apartment had admitted that the girl had been with him since he had picked her up the previous night, she had probably taken the shot while in his apartment. So he couldn't be quite as innocent about how she had died as he claimed to be. Even if he didn't give it to her, she probably took it while she was with him. I sent samples of her blood, liver, bile, stomach contents and urine to the toxicology division and they found traces of quinine, which was sufficient. You don't always find the heroin itself because that may disappear. But the quinine showed that she had died of an acute drug death.

"Three days later I cut myself while doing an autopsy and got serum hepatitis, so I wasn't in the office for quite a while. But I was interested in this case and followed it up when I recovered. It turned out the man had known her for two years. It wasn't a casual pick-up as he had claimed. She used to sleep with him off and on when she wasn't busy with her customers.

"As a result, he was arrested and charged with giving her drugs, but he only got a short jail sentence. He's out now, under surveillance, but probably *still* giving girls drugs. But I haven't been called back to that apartment. Yet."

As this book went to press, Dr. Lehotay was made chief medical examiner of Erie County in 1973, after a struggle of more than two years. This makes her one of the highest ranking female medical detectives in the country.

12

Sexual Asphyxia

The policeman was sure that it was murder when he walked into a bedroom and found a young man of twenty-four sitting up in bed with his hands tied behind his back and a rope around his neck. His mother, who had found him that way, said it was probably suicide, for while he was generally in good spirits, he had been very mysterious about wanting to be alone right before he died. The medical detective who was called to the scene saw that there was padding between the rope and the boy's neck, and that the boy's fly was open, and he immediately concluded that the policeman and the parents of the boy were both wrong, and that the young man had died by accident. Why were the above two clues important, and how did the boy die?

Although the public is generally unaware of the following phenomenon (it has never before been written up in a book for the layman) there is a form of death called by the medical detectives "sexual asphyxia," and by the insurance companies "ritual masturbation." This strange type of asphyxiation occurs when people accidentally strangle or hang themselves while masturbating. It is only in the last decade that medical detectives have come to realize that sexual asphyxia is usually neither a homicide nor suicide, but a strange accident, and the reason for this reevaluation is that at last the cause of these deaths is understood.

People who die from sexual asphyxia apparently become sexually aroused by fantasizing about being tied up. Naturally, this in itself is not dangerous, but they go farther than just thinking about the act and actually bind themselves up, often putting a ligature around their own necks. The first time they do this may only be to dramatize their fantasies of bondage, but they soon learn that compression of the neck enhances the vividness of their images as a result of cerebral anoxia or diminution of oxygen. Then it may become a regular practice, for while in the beginning the noose may only serve as a psychological stimulus, it soon becomes a physiological one as well, for partial unconsciousness may lead to an orgasm.

The reason such people may end up in the offices of the medical detectives when they were merely trying to enjoy themselves is that if they unwittingly apply the pressure on their necks too long or too hard, the blood supply to the brain diminishes and they can totally lose consciousness. Once unconscious, they are unable to remove the ligature to stop the inexorable process and death accidentally may follow.

When a medical detective is called to the scene, and he sees that the person has strangled to death, he searches for clues that indicate whether death was caused by self-imposed asphyxiation, and that the deceased did not commit suicide or fall victim to murder. One way to determine if murder occurred is to see how the person's hands were tied.

Many medical detectives know as much about knots as an old-time sailor, and can tell whether the person could have tied the bonds himself or whether the presence of another person was required. This is not so simple, for some of the knot arrangements people have devised are sometimes so complicated that these deaths were once ascribed to "practicing rock climbing" or "practicing tying of knots." (That seems to be the last thing they were actually practicing.) Furthermore, the situation is sometimes confused if the deceased's hands were tied in back of him in a manner that would seem at first sight difficult, or even impossible, for the person to manage by himself. The medical detectives have seen cases in which the person apparently tied his hands in front of him and then stepped through his hands so they ended up behind him.

The ligature around the person's neck is another giveaway, for there is usually a towel or some form of padding between his neck and the ropes, a padding usually missing in suicide or homicide cases. Padding serves both to prevent marks on the neck (which might cause discomfiting questions about how they got there) and to make the ligature less painful. The presence of padding also helps rule out suicide or homicide, for people who kill themselves or murder others rarely worry about the marks they leave behind—unless they are trying to disguise the cause or manner of death. And people who kill either themselves or others do not go out of their way to ensure a moment of comfort.

Another clue, and perhaps the most important one, is the sexual element that invariably is present in these deaths. If the person is dressed (although often they are not), the genitals are usually exposed; at least the fly is open; semen may be found, or handkerchiefs or tissues nearby to wipe it up. Often pornographic literature or photographs are found (and sometimes books on knot tying), and some of the incredible positions in which these people have been found seem to be inspired by this "literature" since the physical position often matches the open page. While some men blindfold themselves, it is not uncommon for others to arrange mirrors to view the act, or to take pictures for future delectation, little realizing they may not be around to view them.

Elements of fetishism and various perversions are often part of the scene and many of the men are dressed in rubber or leather clothing; others have been found wearing women's underwear or dresses, sometimes with falsies or padded bras. One man was wearing a sanitary napkin; another had attached a metal appliance to himself to allow micturation in the female fashion; and one professional man was found with his testicles tied in back of him so as to simulate the appearance of a female. Although the perversions tend to be heterosexual in nature, phallic objects are sometimes around for anal use. Not surprisingly, whips and belts are likewise found, obviously part of the masochistic fantasy which is reflected also in being bound.

When the above elements are present, a conclusion of sexual asphyxia usually is easy to reach. But variations are harder to classify—or indeed to fathom. For example, people have suffocated accidentally when they put hoods or masks over their faces, and the medical detectives had to analyze the circumstances and decide whether their actions denoted suicidal or sexual purposes. People have died while inhaling chloroform. It is the task of the medical detectives to see whether the deceased seemed to have taken it to heighten his masturbation, which it does, or to end it all, which it can. One man was found hanged with a book open in front of him which said that men always have an erection when they are hanged. The medical detective, Dr. Abraham Rosenthal of Manhattan, had to decide whether the man just wanted to test the theory out a little bit (accidental death) or whether he was determined to come and go at the same time (suicide). He registered it as accidental.

Most victims of sexual asphyxia or its variations are males, usually either in their teens or past fifty, and only one case has been reported in the literature or noted by any of the medical detectives of a female who died from sexual asphyxia. She was nineteen years old and was found dressed as an Oriental harem girl with towels wrapped around her head like a turban. She wore, in addition, a blindfold and gag on her face. The first clue to sexual asphyxia were the ropes tied around her breasts which formed a figure-eight brassiere and looped down around her genitals to stimulate her clitoris. That this arrangement was not an accident, and that the act was clearly sexual, became apparent to the medical detective when he saw pornographic literature in the room (as well as an Alfred Hitchcock suspense story which told of a harem girl who had been tied up in the same manner). Suicide was discounted because she had been in cheerful spirits before she died, and while her mother steadfastly insisted it was homicide and tried to implicate the girl's boyfriend, it was ultimately recognized and registered as an accidental sexual asphyxial death.

There is only one known case of someone who *almost* died from sexual asphyxia and was saved before it was too late. The police once received a report that a woman was seen hanging from a beam in a garage and they raced to the scene to find her unconscious, dressed in black silk stockings, high-heeled shoes, and a girdle. But when they cut her down, they discovered that she was a he. Furthermore, he was absolutely furious and insisted that he had simply been conducting an experiment on the law of gravity.

Before leaving the subject of sexual asphyxia, it should be pointed out that there are accidental asphyxiations that are not sexual in nature. Asphyxiation occurs accidentally with scarves and ties, as happened to dancer Isadora Duncan, whose scarf caught in a moving car. In one gruesome case, a woman on a chair lift at a ski resort was lifted from her chair and hanged by her scarf as it caught on a descending chair. Dr. John Devlin, deputy chief medical examiner of New York City, once had a case in which he was unable to establish the cause of death of a well-dressed businessman. The toxicological report indicated that he had been roaring drunk before he died. Then Dr. Devlin saw that in this man's intoxicated stupor, he simply had leaned his head forward and strangled on his too-tight tie.

Another example of accidental asphyxiation is called "café coronaries." This happens when someone dies by choking on a piece of food, and probably the best known example of this was Tommy Dorsey, who died by choking on food particles while sleeping. The fact that the death was accidental is usually obvious to the medical detectives because the food is often still stuck in the victim's throat at death. But sometimes the piece of food is not gluttonously large or obvious—peanuts can be dangerous, and contrary to popular opinion, oysters *should* be chewed. At times the food particles may be surreptitiously removed by restaurant personnel to avoid any difficulties, especially legal ones.

Sometimes a café coronary can be missed because the person does not always die immediately, but like Dorsey dies hours later when he appears to be completely healthy. That the food is not choking him obviously does not mean that it is not doing so quietly. The people who may have been with the victim while he was eating usually see no connection to the death because it occurs hours later—or perhaps the victim was eating alone and did not mention to anyone his choking, erroneously believing that the food (and crisis) had passed.

Café coronaries have been known for years, while sexual asphyxia has been realized only relatively recently. Of course everyone knows that intercourse, and not just solitary masturbation, has led some people to the medical detectives, but its dangers, especially to those with heart disease, have always been recognized. In fact, Atilla the Hun, who conquered part of the world, was reported to have died from intercourse while conquering just one little woman. In addition, some people have died from fellatio, when one partner strangled on the ejaculate of the other, or died from impaction of the penis in the pharynx. Another danger is strangulation, for the active partner sometimes grasps his partner's neck during intercourse and accidentally chokes him to death.

Only in the last decade, however, has accidental death during masturbation been recognized, and now that the problem finally is understood, it should be taken out of the medical books where it has been closeted and the general public educated to its dangers in hopes of preventing such deaths. One medical detective estimates that sexual asphyxia results in as many as 500 deaths a year in America—and the figure is probably much higher throughout the world.

13

Battered Babies

A mother and father raced to the emergency ward of a hospital at midnight with their dying six-month-old baby. They told the doctor that the infant had fallen out of his stroller that morning and then been bitten by a dog. The next morning the child died. The medical detective found that the baby had a subdural hematoma (bleeding beneath the skull), a fracture of the long bone of his leg, and an earlier fracture, now in a healing phase. In addition, he had several linear abrasions and a circular bite mark. Which seven facts above would make a medical detective suspect that this was a battered baby?

Although the media have been presenting battered babies as a new phenomenon, reflecting our frightening increase in violence, children have been mistreated and mutilated for centuries, and in other countries as well as our own.

The fact that the medical detectives have had to deal with an increasing number of battered children cases, does not mean necessarily that more parents are mistreating their children. It may result from greater awareness of child abuse, resulting in attempts at more accurate reporting of the cause of death, the what-done-it. In the nineteenth as well as the twentieth century, battered children were brought into hospitals and dutifully examined by doctors who diligently published articles on "accident-prone" children who had "vitamin deficiencies" or "bone abnormalities." Only in the last two decades has the cause and extent of the problem been recognized in the United States, though the exact number of children who fall into this category is yet unknown.

It is known that more children under the age of five are killed by their parents than by all diseases combined, and Helfer and Kempe, who wrote the classic medical book on abused children (*The Battered Children*), estimate that a chilling ten to forty thousand children a year are severely battered. Furthermore, one or two children die each day in America from abuse while others are permanently injured or crippled. And of course there are the psychological injuries and their ultimate implications —not only for the victim but for all of society. More than one study has shown that most murderers were severely abused and neglected as children.

Studies on battering parents conflict. Some conclude that there is no apparent pattern in education or socioeconomic status that distinguishes abusing parents, while others find the abusing parents are generally on the lower end of both spectrums. Furthermore, battering is not unique to or concentrated in any one ethnic group, and, in fact, Helfer and Kempe state in *The Battered Child* that abusive parents were not really very different from any picked at random.

Regardless of race, income, or education, however, these parents usually begin to teach their children to fear them (justifiably) when the children are still young. Parents who batter their kids sometimes start when they are two and three weeks old, or when they first have full responsibility for the child, and maltreatment may reach its peak when the child reaches the age of three or four. After some of these parents get through with them, the children are no longer difficult; sometimes they are not even alive. Death may be a relief for them.

When one mother got annoyed with her baby, she placed him on the floor and "kicked him like a football." Another stated nonchalantly that whenever she had trouble getting her child to put on his clothes, she would just twist his arms and legs until he fit into them. The child had fourteen separate injuries to his long bones. Some parents use scalding water to punish, and one mother placed her one-and-a-half-year-old child in a pan of boiling hot water for some minor offense and killed him. A mother gave her two-year-old an enema with scalding water to punish him—an operation that damaged the infant's colon and required a colostomy to repair. Another mother tied a ligature around her son's penis to prevent him from urinating so she wouldn't have to clean his diapers so often. He developed gangrene of the genitals.

Some parents are not actually battering, they simply are neglecting their children, but if continued long enough and carried to a sufficient degree, the results can be equally damaging. For example, parents who rarely change their children's diapers or bedding can cause them to contract such a severe case of diaper rash that the skin of their genitalia and perineum become denuded. If this is continued long enough, the child can suffer a permanent loss of pigment in the area and the skin around the sexual and excretory organs of black children may even turn white.

The overt reasons that the parents give for punishing their children are often as trivial as the crime is heinous. Dr. Lester Adelson, medical examiner of Cleveland, reports that one mother killed her three-and-a-half-year-old child by unscrewing a pepper shaker and forcing the entire contents of the bottle down his mouth to punish him for taking the nursing bottle away from his thirteen-month-old sibling. Another mother, who killed her two-year-old child by burning and beating him, said she did it because she resented the fact that he needed attention. Some parents may mean well, but batter their children in a misguided attempt to instill obedience. One father said that if his child did not come immediately when he called, he gave him a "gentle tug on the ear" as a reminder. In the name of obedience the child's ear was partially torn away from his head. Another father honestly believed that by being "strict," as he put it, he was bringing his child up to obey and respect the law. He saw no incongruity in talking about teaching obedience to the law while *he* was in jail for child battering.

Of course, the underlying causes of abuse are a different matter. Many of these parents were battered children themselves, and while some were not physically abused, they were all emotionally battered. Another reason for their behavior seems to be downright ignorance and lack of understanding of what a child can and cannot comprehend. One mother started slapping her child at the age of three weeks to teach him not to reach for a spoon, and she simply did not understand that a child that age cannot control his hand movements, nor can he comprehend the relation between the punishment and his offense. Brandt F. Steele and Carl B. Pollock, psychiatrists at the University of Colorado School of Medicine, who have studied battering parents, have found that these parents commonly expect and demand a great deal from their children and consistently treat them as older than they really are.

Other parents beat their children because they believe that the children are there to satisfy *their* desires, and since they are basically children themselves, they resent the dependency of their infants. Many psychiatrists have noticed this role reversal as the parents look to the child for nurture and protection. One mother said: "I waited so long to have my baby and when she came she never did anything for me." Some parents take the fact that their child does not do anything for them as a rejection. One mother said of her three-month-old (then in the hospital recovering from his battering): "I have never felt really loved all my life. When the baby was born, I thought it would love me, but when he cried all the time, it meant he didn't love me so I hit him."

While some parents single out one child for battering, others spare none of them. (One study in the *British Medical Journal* showed that if one child was battered, there was a thirteen to one chance that another in the family would also be injured.) Some parents murder more than one child and in one morgue the receptionist recognized the father who had come to identify his eighteen-month-old baby, dead from battering, because he had been there a month earlier to identify an older son who died from the same thing.

Similarly, the woman who killed her child with pepper had been tried three years earlier for neglecting another child in the family, who was then two and a half months old. She had been acquitted. One of her children had been blinded in one eye when she threw a bottle at him, and even the infant killed by the pepper had a fractured leg, which the mother claimed came from a fall.

Battering parents usually lie to doctors about the cause of their child's injuries. It is the job of the doctor, therefore, to recognize when a child's injuries result from child abuse rather than from whatever reasons the parents may give, and to report the parents before the child is killed. However, the discovery sometimes must come from the medical examiner. Even then it is not too late to report it, not only in order to punish the parents, but to save any other children in the house.

Many clues show whether the child is suffering or died from battering. One is to note when the parents first went to get help. Most parents will immediately seek aid for a sick child, but battering parents may wait for hours, even days, before taking their child to the hospital even for a major injury. The injuries themselves are a good indication of battering, for subdural hematomas, bruises, fractures, and separations of the long bones—common because these parents frequently use the child's arms and legs as handles with which to yank him—are signs of abuse. Moreover, X-rays often reveal bone injuries in various stages of healing, and this is another strong sign of battering, which is defined as *repetitive* mistreatment.

Bruises can be a good indication of battering, especially if they leave a mark in the same shape as the object that caused them. Belt buckles, rulers, electric cords, irons, cigarettes, fists—all favorite weapons of assaultive parents—sometimes leave as distinctive an outline on the child as if they were painted on. When these patterned bruises are evident, they often tell the real story—unlike the parents. One mother told a medical detective that her three-year-old had "banged his head on the floor," but he had loop and linear abrasions on his body that were clearly in the shape of the cord and the ruler with which he was hit.

Another sign that the parents are hiding something is the number of bruises the child sustains. One mother insisted that her child fell from his stroller and caught his ear on the handle, but he had *three* injuries on his face, all supposedly from one fall to the floor. Still another clue to battering is the unlikeliness of the parents' story, such as that of the obviously kicked child whose mother claimed he "fell and caught his stomach against the door."

In addition to determining whether a child died of battering, the medical detectives often help the police establish the who-done-it—that is, which parent killed the child. They cannot allow the appearance or general impression of the parents to be their guide, and in fact, one study showed that the parent who gave the impression of being normal and innocent was often the guilty one. Medical evidence often is their guide. Even if the parents do not tell which one did the battering, the bruises sometimes do. Fractures and bruises requiring considerable force are usually inflicted by the father. The size of the bruise can be matched with the parent's fists to see which made the blow. The size of teeth from bite marks have also been matched to the parents, for it is not uncommon for these parents to bite their children, like the animals they really are.

In one case, a dead child was brought into the morgue with bruises and bite marks that might have been inflicted by any of four people in his family: the father, the stepmother, or the two remaining children. To digress for a moment, Dr. Lester Adelson, the forensic pathologist of Cuyahoga County (who now works for Dr. Gerber), has found that some murderers of infants turn out to be children themselves, and he coined the term "battering child" to describe these homicidal youngsters. In one of his cases, the attending physician concluded that the infant had "strangled on milk" (*sic*), but Dr. Adelson discovered during the autopsy that she had been murdered, and the perpetrator later turned out to be her eight-year-old retarded sister. Dr. Adelson found five more similar cases in his area, in which the victim, under a year old, had been killed by siblings ranging from two to eight years old, always with jealousy as the motive. But in the case above, the size of the teeth marks immediately ruled out the children.

When one of the neighbors told the police that she had seen the father hit his children, he was arrested. In order to eliminate the stepmother as a suspect, the police took the woman's dental impressions. But when the tooth sleuth, Dr. Lowell Levine, forensic medical consultant, looked at her dental impressions, he discovered that *she* was the one who had bitten and battered the baby to death, since her teeth marks matched those on the baby's body.

Some people believe that with the increased use of contraception and legal abortions battering will decrease, since fewer unwanted children will be brought into this world. Others, more pessimistic, believe that the population growth as well as an increasing acceptance of violence in our society will lead to even more cases of abuse. Some solutions are being tried. In Los Angeles a Mothers Anonymous has been instituted for battering parents, which, in addition to group therapy and intervention by other parents at times of stress, allows battering parents temporarily to exchange children when they feel they are going to lose control. Similar groups are spreading to other U.S. cities as well; in New York it is called Parents Anonymous, to include abusive fathers as well. In New Jersey, hot lines have been established to handle reports of child abuse even after regular working hours. And many states now make it mandatory for doctors to report suspected child abuse cases.

One way to reduce the number of deaths from beating would be for every doctor to become a bit of a medical detective, looking for signs of battering whenever he examines an injured child. Unfortunately, many private doctors are reluctant to make accusations. They hesitate to ask their clients to pay for X-rays which the courts may use as evidence against them. Hospitals also fail to recognize the symptoms because rarely do battered children come to the same hospital twice. The parents usually take the child to a different hospital each time they injure him in order to avoid suspicion. And even when the doctors and hospitals recognize the problem, the agencies responsible often fail to do anything about it. And when agencies *do* try to take the child away from his parents, and give the parents what they really deserve, prosecution is difficult, usually resulting in probation or short prison sentences. Most depressing, many of these parents who are caught, and sometimes even convicted of child battering, are pregnant again at the time.

In the opening case, the seven points that suggest a battered baby are: 1) the parents waited nearly twelve hours before bringing the child to the hospital at midnight; 2) the story that the child fell out of his stroller and was bitten by a dog sounds far-fetched; 3) a subdural hematoma (bleeding beneath the skull) plus a fracture of the long bone of the leg are often the result of battering; 4) there were signs of an earlier fracture; 5) a fall would probably not produce a linear abrasion of that sort; 6) the child had several linear abrasions from only one alleged fall; 7) the bite marks of dogs are U-shaped whereas this one was circular.

PART IV

THE MEDICAL DETECTIVES

14

Dr. Milton Helpern: "The Chief"

Obviously, the medical examiner in charge of all the murders in Manhattan—*plus* the suicides, accidents, and natural deaths that fall under his jurisdiction—must be a busy and competent person. Such a man is Dr. Milton Helpern, affectionately known by the people who work for him as "The Chief." Dr. Helpern, who is seventy years old and has been with the Office for more than forty years, has been New York City's chief medical examiner since 1954. He has performed personally more than 20,000 autopsies, witnessed 40,000 more, and as *The New York Times* said, "knows more about violent death than anyone in the country."

Dr. Helpern is one of the authors of the 1,500-page bible of forensic medicine, *Legal Medicine, Pathology and Toxicology*. He has been a medical witness more than 3,000 times, presents almost 100 lectures a year, teaches at three medical schools, belongs to forty professional groups, and is president or past president of five. In fact, his full list of credits and qualifications is so long and so impressive that when he takes the witness stand, it is common for the defense attorney to "magnanimously" offer to waive this part of the testimony. (The prosecution usually objects, of course, since it wants the jury to hear it.)

Dr. Helpern has a staff of almost 150 people, and in addition he receives free full-time help from an extremely capable assistant—his wife. Helpern likes to say of Beatrice Helpern, who works with him at the New York Medical Examiner's Office at Thirtieth Street and First Avenue, "Some women become secretaries so they can marry the boss, but she married the boss and became a secretary." Still, there is one thing that Mrs. Helpern does not do, and that is accompany him on cases. According to writer Martha Weinman Lear, only once did Mrs. Helpern go along on a homicide case, and she was appalled at the filth and blood all around. When she saw her husband casually touch the body, she couldn't stand it. "*Please*, put on some gloves," she cried. Her husband turned to her: "This is the last time you're ever coming with me." And it was.

Helpern, therefore, goes out on his cases alone, or else he works downstairs in the autopsy room, or in his first-floor office, a large room with close to fifty diplomas lining the wall plus thousands and thousands of slides representing the extraordinary cases he has handled. Talking to many medical examiners is a funny thing. After a while you hear the same type of who-done-it stories repeatedly and it is often easy to guess the ending before it comes. For example, the medical detective will say, "So I was told it was a natural death but I immediately noticed this cherry-red lividity . . ." ("Carbon monoxide poisoning," I interrupt.) "Okay, now let me tell you about the time I was told this little child had fallen out of her stroller but I saw a subdural hematoma . . ." ("A battered baby," I say.) But talking to Dr. Helpern about his cases is fascinating because they *really* are different, and he has caught things that not only a forensic medicine buff would miss, but probably most other medical detectives in this country. (Some are chronicled in Marshall Houts' biography of Helpern, *Where Death Delights.*)

Take, for example, one of his "typical" battered baby cases. The child was brought to him with severe damage to the liver and the parents asserted that they did not know how it happened—which was suspicious. He brings out the slide of the bruised liver—obviously a battered baby—until he points out that there is no hemorrhage there. The liver had been bruised *after* death and it was the hospital nurses, not the parents, who were accidentally responsible. The child had died a natural death and in their attempts to resuscitate him, they had damaged his liver.

Or take his "easy," clear-cut strangulation case, which started when a drunk called the police to report that he had been drinking and fighting with his common-law wife and had finally strangled her to death. When her body was brought to Dr. Helpern, it was a reversal of the usual medical detective tale of he-said-she-died-from-a-fall-but-I-saw-she-had-petechial-hemorrhages. Helpern saw that she had *no* petechial hemorrhages and, in fact, no signs of asphyxiation whatsoever. When he performed the autopsy, he discovered that she had died naturally from cirrhosis of the liver. When the police told this to the husband, he still steadfastly stuck to his story of strangulation and no one knew (or knows) whether he was lying, insane, or had dreamt the whole thing. The case was dismissed in court, however, after Helpern proved that the man could not have been directly responsible for her death regardless of what he insisted. The man walked out free. Two weeks later he committed suicide.

Dr. Helpern has a so-then-I-noticed-a-cherry-pink-lividity-and-knew-he-died-from-carbon-monoxide story, but here too it is unusual. Yes, carbon monoxide poisoning was the ultimate cause of death, the what-done-it, but attempts had been made to kill this derelict by feeding him over a period of time more than three gallons of automobile antifreeze in his drinks, along with a can of decayed sardines with the tin from the can shred into it, plus diseased oysters and clams. When that failed to kill him, the group of bums attempting murder tried removing his clothes and leaving him outside in sub-zero weather, first pouring gallons of ice water on him, and when he survived that as well, they pushed him in front of a fast-moving car. Finally they accomplished their goal by getting him to pass out and then putting the gas hose directly in his mouth—all to collect his insurance.

Another off-beat case started in the autopsy room when the typical report on a normal white person began, "This is the body of a well-developed, well-nourished white female . . ." There was only one problem. Helpern noticed that despite the brunette's shapely figure and her lovely feminine face, the nipples of the well-proportioned breasts were too small for a female. He soon found that under each breast ran a transverse scar showing she had had her breasts built up with plastic surgery, and he saw that the penis had been removed, the scrotum made into a labia major, a small vagina constructed, and the testicles placed inside the body. So, "This is the body of a well-developed, well-nourished, white *male* . . ."

She (he) had died of an overdose of drugs. A young

man, Mr. X, and his friend, Miss Y, arrived to identify the body. The effeminate Mr. X turned out to be the brother of the deceased, and Helpern noticed that Miss Y's pupils were constricted, suggesting that she was on drugs just as her dead friend had been. When he asked Miss Y to tell him more about the operation that the woman (man) in the autopsy room had undergone, Miss Y said that *she* too had had the operation and had once been a man. Afterward, the two "girls" became roommates, Greenwich Village entertainers, and prostitutes.

Six months later, Dr. Helpern's secretary called him to say that Miss Y was back and Helpern wondered aloud what on earth she had come to speak to him about. But the secretary explained that she wasn't there to see him. She was "on the table downstairs—dead." Helpern, remembering her constricted pupils on that earlier visit, looked for needle marks and, sure enough, found fresh ones. She, too, had died from drugs.

The next day a woman came to identify the body and while Helpern did not remember meeting her, she was insistent that they had met before. It turned out she was the former *Mr.* X, who had undergone the same operation, and she (he) was the sister (brother) of the first dead woman (man).

The job of the chief medical examiner is never dull. And never is it unimportant. Dr. Helpern not only finds out why people die, but saves others who might have died of the same cause by discovering and publicizing the cause of death and working to get laws enacted that would prevent them from recurring. For he takes very seriously the Latin motto in the Medical Examiner's Office: "This is the Place where Death Delights to Help the Living."

15

Dr. Thomas Noguchi: "My Schedule Is Murder"

A lot of people in Los Angeles literally were getting away with murder before Dr. Thomas Noguchi became the coroner-medical examiner of Los Angeles, California. Before he took over, most of the autopsies were being handled by medical students who were assigned six to eight bodies for each eight-hour shift. Naturally, they could not perform autopsies on all those people in that short space of time, so they would look for any sign that indicated that a death might be due to natural causes and then so attribute it. The danger inherent in this situation became obvious when a ninety-seven-year-old woman with petechial hemorrhages, suggesting strangulation, was found to have clogged coronary arteries and the death was ascribed to the latter. A year later, someone came forward and said he had strangled her to death.

Dr. Thomas Noguchi was the first Oriental-American in California to be made a county department head. He was appointed to the job only after six weeks of bitter arguments between the Civil Service and the medical authorities which represented the California medical schools. The latter claimed Noguchi at age forty was too young and relatively inexperienced to become part of their faculty, as is standard for the chief coroner-medical examiner in Los Angeles. But his problems really began only after he got his job. Six months after his appointment he was summarily dismissed, accused of saying, for example, that he could "perform an autopsy on the living" (in reference to someone he did not like), that he hoped Robert Kennedy would die or a 747 would crash in Los Angeles because then he (Noguchi) would become famous.

Dr. Noguchi was given a hearing, after which he was cleared fully of all the charges against him, reinstated, and given all the back pay that had been kept from him. Even then, his problems were not over, and his office underwent additional embarrassment when the newspapers reported that the doctor immediately under him was not a licensed doctor. He had taken all the courses, but had neglected to take the final exams. Noguchi refused to comment, but the situation may have brought him some personal satisfaction since the so-called doctor had been the primary witness against Noguchi at his hearing.

Dr. Noguchi does not mind talking about his hearing (he brings up his dismissal before his interviewers do), and he does not object to talking about some of his more famous cases. His first one was in August of 1962, when he was sent to investigate the death of Marilyn Monroe. So unexpected was her death to him (and to the country) that until he got there, he thought it was someone who had the same name as the famous actress. ("Her face looked very peaceful, although it may have been because the muscles relax after death.") He also did the six-hour autopsy on Robert Kennedy, and concluded that death came from pressure on the brain stem due to swelling of the brain and bleeding. Jimi Hendrix and Janis Joplin were two other cases ("They had very used bodies, reflecting the hard lives they lived"), and one of the most difficult (and sensational) was the Sharon Tate murder case.

After Noguchi witnessed the gruesome scene at the Tate home, he had to examine, analyze, and list more than 100 stab and gunshot wounds plus blows from a blunt instrument. One victim alone (Voityck Frykowski) was stabbed fifty-one times, shot twice, and struck thirteen times on the head. Each of seven stab wounds could have been the cause of his death, and this was true for some of the others, for three of the victims together had seventeen stab wounds, each of which could have been fatal. Noguchi also had to figure out why one of the victims had five wounds although she had only been shot four times, and he concluded that the bullet that went through her left arm then went on into her chest.

In that case, and others, he did not mind using a slightly unconventional approach, and he appointed a team of forensic psychologists and psychiatrists to study the bizarre scene to try to determine who might have done it. They concluded that it was not the work of one person, but that two or three people were probably involved, that one of the killers was paranoid, and that one was a female. Some of his unconventional investigation he claims is simply "common sense method," as, for example, when he determined the time of death by examining the amount of chlorophyl in the grass underneath the deceased. Another time he used the common sense method was when a man was found dead in his car at the bottom of a canyon. He appeared to have killed himself with a bullet through his head, but no gun could be found, which meant it could have been a homicide instead. Rather than simply gathering clues at the autopsy, Noguchi went back to the scene with the police and checked the tire marks of the car. He saw several yards of the same tire pattern on the winding road, and noted that the pattern suddenly swerved. Noguchi told the police to look for the gun in that area, and they found it within a few yards. Noguchi explains that the man had probably been driving with the left window down, shot himself, and because of the winding road and recoil action of the gun, the gun fell out of the window before the car went down the canyon.

Such investigations obviously take time, and Noguchi may take six hours to ten days before coming to a conclusion about a case. ("The body is not going anyplace anyway," he says.) This reflects his great involvement with his work. In fact, he seems always to be working, and he admits that, for example, if he is shopping and sees a hammer in a carpentry shop, he will examine it from the standpoint of what kind of a mark it would leave on a person's head. In his spare time he reads mystery stories, and is a friend of such as Erle Stanley Gardner, who, according to *Esquire*, once called Noguchi and said, "A man finds a petrified finger. Go with it."

Despite his long working hours, however, he tries not to get emotionally involved in his cases: "The coroner is the one person who must be stable during death. I cannot break down and cry over each case." In his attempt to maintain objectivity, unlike some medical detectives he will not autopsy friends or relatives. His detachment is not always successful, however, and he admits that he gets very upset over battered children cases, such as the time a child was brought to him with over 300 bruises that obviously had been inflicted over a long period of time.

The cases of the medical detectives are basically

similar throughout the country, although Noguchi says that some Los Angeles murders show great imagination and sophistication. Because the area is so vast, the killer usually has to travel to his victim and must, therefore, plan in advance. The most commonly used weapons are the "Saturday night special" (22-caliber gun), tire irons, and blunt instruments related to cars (such as jacks). The month of December sees the largest number of homicides (as well as of suicides and traffic deaths based on alcohol) and this differs from killings in wintery New York, where the citizens seem to wait for summer to release their homicidal aggressions. Still, the work of the medical detectives out West does not differ much from that in the East; most medical detectives agree that the work now being done in Los Angeles is good.

So does Dr. Noguchi. While he was on the Dick Cavett show, Cavett asked him, "With your medical knowledge, could you commit an undetectable murder?" Noguchi explained that different jurisdictions handle cases differently, "but I would be very careful if I were going to commit a murder in Los Angeles now," he said confidently.

16

Dr. Cyril Wecht: Mysteries of the JFK Assassination

The following is not an attempt to show whether President Kennedy was shot from the sixth floor of the Texas School Book Depository or from elsewhere, as many have stated. It is simply a presentation of the medical evidence in the assassination with both known and recent findings included. The purpose of the chapter is to shed some light on how medical detectives handle bullet wound cases, to show how incredibly complicated they can be even when they involve (probably) only two bullets, to show how one such autopsy was conducted, what the findings were, what mistakes were made, and what another medical detective, Dr. Cyril Wecht, has concluded from the same material.

It is now almost a decade since the thirty-fifth president of the United States was assassinated, and after all this time, what is surprising is not just that so many questions have remained unanswered, but that so many official "answers" have remained unquestioned. Every time a new fact emerges, we learn that not everything told before was true; more to the point, we learn that we have not been told everything.

The most recent analysis of the Kennedy assassination was made by Dr. Cyril Wecht, a medical detective who is the coroner of Pittsburgh and Allegheny County in Pennsylvania. Dr. Wecht is past president of the American Academy of Forensic Sciences and the American College of Legal Medicine, and has had experience with some 1,500 gunshot wounds and deaths in his eleven years as a medical detective. World-wide headlines trumpeted his discovery that Kennedy's brain had disappeared. But other findings at the National Archives were equally troubling.

Dr. Wecht was the first critic of the Warren Commission, i.e., the first believer in a conspiracy theory to be allowed to analyze the sixty-nine autopsy photographs and X-rays of Kennedy, the bullets and other material relating to the assassination; and he is convinced that what he saw at the National Archives still "proves a conspiracy." Not everyone agrees—and some medical detectives criticize him for making such public statements. Still, one cannot easily dismiss his findings, for Wecht is not only a doctor *and* a lawyer, but also a specialist in forensic pathology, all of which are basic to a re-creation of the JFK assassination.

As a rule, medical detectives have no problems in gunshot cases in determining the what-done-it. It is usually obvious, although sometimes a gunshot wound in the head may be so well hidden by the hair and bleed so little that the cause of death may not be realized immediately. More often, the detectives find difficulty in determining the how-was-it-done, that is, whether the death was homicidal, suicidal, or accidental. Even when both the cause and the method of death are known, however, as in the Kennedy case, the medical detectives are often called upon to provide collateral information, such as where the bullets entered and exited, their exact location, and their paths through the body, all of which can be crucial to the re-creation of the crime.

In the Kennedy assassination, the official Warren Commission report gave the following sequence of events. Kennedy, traveling along Elm Street, was shot from behind by Lee Harvey Oswald, who was standing on the sixth floor of the Texas School Book Depository. The Commission held that this was an isolated instance of assassination—not a conspiracy enacted by more than one man.

According to the Warren Commission, three shots were fired. The first entered Kennedy's back and exited at his throat, at which point they said it may have ricocheted and wounded Governor Connally. The second and fatal bullet entered and smashed the brain. The third shot was unaccounted for, and still remains a mystery.

But other theories abound, and not even the Warren Commission put them to rest. The most prevalent asserts that a party of assassins planned the murder: that Kennedy was shot from the front, that Connally was hit by a different bullet, and that the evidence was misconstrued or even maliciously and purposefully misrepresented for unknown reasons.

Actually, the questions of where the bullets entered and exited Kennedy's body, their exact locations, and how many there were are the important questions of the JFK assassination, for all the theories of all those people supposedly seen doing all that shooting from all those angles are simply conjecture. What really matters is whether there is physical evidence to show that all the bullets entered Kennedy's body from behind (where the

Texas School Book Depository was located) and above (the sixth-floor window), and how many bullets lodged in him.

The first question concerns where each bullet entered and exited. It is not difficult for the medical detectives to determine whether a bullet wound is one of entrance or exit: the wound created by a bullet as it enters the body is usually smaller than the hole it makes on leaving. In fact, sometimes the entrance wound is even smaller than the bullet itself, because the human skin, being extremely elastic, tries to return to its original closed condition after being penetrated by a bullet. The exit wound is usually the larger of the two because as the bullet rips through the body, it tears apart the tissues in its path, pushing the tissue along with and in front of it.

As it happened, the three doctors who performed the autopsy on Kennedy were Commander James J. Humes, Commander J. Thornton Boswell, and Lieutenant-Colonel Pierre Finck. Yet despite the fact that they all came from the armed forces, none had much experience with bullet wounds. None apparently realized that a standard procedure when performing an autopsy on a body that has recently undergone surgery (as did Kennedy when he was raced to the Dallas hospital) requires checking with the surgeons to find out what they did.

Since the medical detectives did not call the surgeons, they did not know that there was a bullet wound in Kennedy's throat as well as in his back—the Dallas surgeons had obliterated this orifice when they performed a tracheotomy on Kennedy in a futile attempt to resuscitate him. Inasmuch as evidence of the frontal bullet wound was "gone," the medical detectives thought that the only body wound was in Kennedy's back. They therefore concluded that it was one of entrance *and* exit, and that the bullet had penetrated Kennedy from the back and then turned around in a circle or fallen out in what they admitted was "a rather inexplicable fashion."

Although the surgeons, in utilizing the bullet hole for the tracheotomy, had made a wise decision medically, the unfortunate result was not only to confuse the autopsy doctors, but also to change the size and characteristics of the throat wound, so that it was impossible, even after the autopsy was completed (when the medical examiners learned of the tracheotomy), to reexamine the wounds and compare their characteristics in order to determine the entry wound. Neither could the Dallas surgeons make the comparison, for just as the medical detectives had never seen the wound in the throat, so the surgeons had not seen the one in his back, never having turned Kennedy over. So the three medical examiners came to the conclusion that the wound in the president's back was "presumably of entrance."

Yet, it is possible that this conclusion was wrong, for the size of the back wound apparently was larger than that in the throat. This has been determined by querying each group of doctors independently.

The Dallas surgeons who saw the throat wound at the operation described it as from three to five millimeters, or about one-fifth of an inch in diameter; extremely small. The autopsy doctors described the wound in Kennedy's back as from four to seven millimeters, which certainly appears to be larger than the three to five millimeters given for the exit wound in the front. Was the wound in the back, then, actually an exit wound?

Now, it sometimes does happen that the entrance wound is larger than the exit wound, but it is not common. Josiah Thompson, author of *Six Seconds in Dallas*, cites medical evidence to show that one bullet entered Kennedy's back, and that the small front neck wound came from a fragment of bone which exited from Kennedy's throat as a result of the second bullet. Dr. Wecht feels that it is highly possible that Kennedy's throat wound is really an entrance wound, and he notes that the back wound that he examined in the autopsy photographs had some characteristics of an exit wound. If so, it could mean that Kennedy was shot from the front, as well as from the rear.

One way to determine whether or not that first shot came from the sixth floor of the Texas School Book Depository is to determine its angle of trajectory. This can be done by comparing the location of the two wounds, back and throat, for if the assassin was at the sixth-floor window (where Oswald was said to have stood), shooting at the president's back, then the wound in the back probably would be higher than the one in the front. According to the FBI, the downward angle should be at least 17 degrees. And basically, this is what the autopsy reported, but the problem is that the actual *pictures* of Kennedy drawn at the autopsy by one of the doctors before a "team meeting" was held to decide what the autopsy report should say, placed that back wound four inches *lower* than where it was placed in the (later) written report. If the picture is correct, it means that the bullet appears to have entered from a point lower than where it exited, which is a pretty neat trick for someone shooting from six floors above.

Now, it may have been just an honest error made by a group of men who had had very little experience with bullet wounds. But Dr. Wecht argues that the locations of everything else (such as birthmarks and scars) were correctly drawn. Moreover, it would be extremely difficult for even a layman, not to mention three doctors, to make such an egregious error. It is true that one could miscalculate a point on someone's back by four inches, but Dr. Wecht notes that the discrepancy between the two locations of the bullet wound is more glaring because in their report these doctors placed their bullet wound in the wrong part of the body. They said the wound was at the nape of the neck, when the diagrams drawn at the autopsy placed it down in the back. It is hard to believe that three top doctors could not distinguish between someone's neck and his back.

So where was the bullet hole really? Which do we believe? The bullet hole in Kennedy's jacket conformed to the picture: in other words, it was in his back, four inches below his neck, four inches lower than the position stated in the written report. The defenders of the Warren Commission report say, however, that Kennedy's jacket bunched up as he waved to the crowds, riding up onto his neck, although photographs refute the idea. So if the jacket did bunch and the autopsy doctors decided where Kennedy was shot by looking for the bullet wound in the jacket—which is unheard of since one performs an autopsy on a body, not a jacket—then such a mistake could be plausible.

The placement of the bullet wound in the nape of the neck—higher than the exit wound—may not be a mistake. The throat wound may only *appear* to be higher than the one in back due to an interesting anatomical fact first noted in this connection not by a doctor but by a lawyer. Professor John Kaplan of Stanford University explains that the lowest part of your neck in front is further down than the lowest part of your neck in the back. (Feel it; it's true.) He argues that Kennedy was shot in the nape of the neck, and since the bullet was traveling at a downward angle, it still emerged from the lower front neck.

A few theorists have argued, on the other hand, that Kennedy was shot in the back and that the bullet somehow ricocheted upward inside the body. This is wrong, for the bullet hit nothing inside the body to bounce off of.

Others have insisted that the shot emerged at what appeared to be an upward angle because Kennedy was leaning forward. However the photographs and films of the assassination do not confirm this. In fact, Kennedy never fell far forward even immediately after the second shot, because due to his back problems, he was wearing a canvas brace with metal stays together with an Ace bandage with extra padding. Indeed this brace is what killed him, because it held him totally rigid. Had he been able to fall forward from that first shot, he might have been saved, since that second fatal bullet came within millimeters of missing him anyway.

In addition to the small size of the throat's "exit wound" (suggestive of an entrance wound) and the angle of fire (suggestive of a shot from an angle lower than a sixth-floor window above and in back of him) there is further evidence to show that Kennedy may have been shot from the right front, perhaps where the Grassy Knoll was located. All the doctors in Dallas who saw Kennedy thought that his massive head wound, caused by the second bullet, had been inflicted by a bullet which came from the right.

The theory is supported by the film taken by an observer, Abraham Zapruder. It clearly shows that as Kennedy was struck by the second fatal shot, he moved backward and to the left—a strange movement to make if he was shot from behind, considering the impact of the heavy (160-grain), high-speed (2,200-feet-per-second), military bullet. None of the explanations offered for Kennedy's backward and leftward movement seem valid, for the films show that his head struck nothing, that his wife did not touch him, and that the car did not accelerate for three more seconds; and several doctors believe that the small time factor (fifty-six milliseconds) between the moment of impact of the bullet and the commencement of the backward movement makes a physiological opisthotonus-like reaction unlikely.

In addition, many experts have criticized the Warren Commission's single-bullet theory. This theory states that the first bullet entered Kennedy's back and exited through his neck, then proceeded to strike Connally in the back, wrist, and thigh. Those who know nothing about the meanderings of bullets have dismissed this as inherently preposterous. But actually, bullets have ended up in surprising places, as one man learned when he attempted suicide by shooting himself in the heart, and woke up ten days later in the hospital to find the bullet lodged in his scrotum. The explanation for this (and the reason that about half of all the people who try to shoot themselves through the heart miss) is that when a bullet strikes bone (in that case the breastbone), it may deflect. The Warren Commission claimed that this is what happened to that first bullet, but this is unlikely because the bullet that passed through Kennedy's neck did not strike any bones. It went cleanly through Kennedy, and then for some inexplicable reason veered right and struck Connally in three places. Even Connally, who had time to turn around after he heard the first shot, said it was "inconceivable" to him that he had been struck by the same bullet that hit Kennedy.

Another thing that makes it difficult to accept this single-bullet theory is the heavy weight of the bullet after it allegedly did all of this damage. By comparing the mean weight of several bullets, experts established that this one weighed 160–61 grams before it was fired. After traveling through seven layers of skin (which offers a great deal of resistance) plus two large bones (Connally's rib and wrist), it weighed almost the same—158.6 grams. Furthermore, the bullet was in practically perfect condition, with its lands and grooves miraculously intact save for some slight flattening on the bottom third of the bullet. "It looked as if a strong man had squeezed it," says Dr. Wecht. So pristine was the bullet, in fact, that many people, adherents to the conspiracy theory, suspected that the bullet was deposited carefully at the scene of the assassination.

There are two ways to test the validity of this single-bullet theory and to see whether all the bullets and fragments that were found really came from the same gun—Oswald's. Yet the results of neither of these tests are available. The first is a neutron activation analysis (such as the FBI made with the hair in the Cincinnati Strangler case). But this was never done. Another test is the spectrographic analysis done on all the recovered metal fragments. This was performed, but the results of this test have never been released, and Dr. Wecht discovered that this report too is missing from the National Archives.

Another way to determine whether one bullet hit both Connally and Kennedy would have been to examine Connally's suit at the point where the bullet penetrated. When a bullet is released from a gun it has lubricating grease on it from the barrel. If the bullet had gone through Kennedy's body, however, the grease would have been wiped clean and also there would have been no trace elements from metallic particles. (Conversely, if grease were present on Connally's suit, then the bullet could not have gone through Kennedy first.) Yet, Dr. Wecht discovered that while Kennedy's clothes were examined immediately after the assassination, Connally's were analyzed only after his suit had already been dry-cleaned and his shirt laundered, and by then any grease and metallic particles were gone.

Although critics of the Warren Commission have made this single-bullet theory a major issue to support a conspiracy—and they may well be right in saying that the Warren Commission probably erred on this point—it does not follow necessarily that more than two killers were involved. This implausible single-bullet theory originally was formulated because it was believed that Kennedy could not have been shot between frames 166 and 210 on the Zapruder film, at which time Oswald's view was hidden by the foliage of an oak tree. Yet Kennedy had to have been shot before frame 225, since he was then already visibly reacting from the first shot. Thus, it was deduced he was shot between frames 210 and 225.

Opinions vary only slightly about when Connally was hit. It is always placed between frames 230 and 238, and there is no dispute that the last and fatal shot hit Kennedy at frame 313.

In order to see how long it would take to fire three shots from a Mannlicher-Carcano rifle such as Oswald allegedly used, a sharpshooter shot three bullets from the same type of rifle. It took him 4.6 seconds. The minimum amount of time, therefore, in which Oswald could have fired and reloaded that rifle twice was 2.3 seconds. This comes to exactly forty frames on the Zapruder film. If

Kennedy was hit after frame 210, Connally could not have been shot between frames 230 and 238 by the same gun. The argument goes that either there were two assassins, or else Connally was struck by the same bullet as Kennedy, and since the Warren Commission ruled out a second assassin, it had to hold to the single-bullet theory.

It should be pointed out that Kennedy could have been shot *before* frame 210, when it was said that Oswald's view of Kennedy was hidden by the oak tree. Actually Oswald's view was obscured only partially by that tree. Marshall Houts in *Where Death Delights* notes that when the assassination was reenacted, it took place in the month of May, although the actual assassination had occurred in *November*, when the foliage of that tree would have been different. So there actually may have been time for one sharpshooter to hit Kennedy, Connally, and then Kennedy again; in which case the Warren Commission might never have had to adopt the controversial single-bullet theory.

In addition to all the technical questions raised by the assassination, Dr. Wecht raised questions recently about some of the other things he saw at the National Archives. Dr. Wecht made it clear before he got to the National Archives that he wanted to examine the brain or the slides of the brain taken at a supplementary autopsy two weeks after the first autopsy, and after the brain had hardened in formalin. ("I didn't want an issue; I wanted the brain.") The brain is important in determining the direction of the second bullet, which is still in dispute, as well as the number of bullets that struck him. To determine the path of the bullet the medical detectives can examine the tissues nearby, for bullets burn and soil tissues around the point of entry, but not at the point of exit. But as stated, the brain has disappeared.

While it is generally common to dispose of a brain after the supplementary autopsy, to do so in this case is strange. As Dr. Wecht states: "Who would take the responsibility for destroying a president's brain?" Furthermore, he knows that the brain was still in existence one and a half years after Kennedy's death, for it was listed in a memorandum of transfer from Admiral Burkley, Kennedy's personal physician, to the National Archives when Burkley sent over all the autopsy materials. Incidentally, microscopic autopsy slides which also would show the burning and soiling at the entrance site of the wounds also have disappeared.

While slides of the brain have disappeared, however, there remain large photographs of Kennedy's brain. In the anterior portion of the right cerebral hemisphere of the brain in one photo, Dr. Wecht saw a dark brownish-black object which in a few places has a white glistening effect. It appeared to be about thirteen by twenty millimeters (approximately one-half by three-fourths of an inch), although it may be larger than in the photograph, since the additional brain mass around it hides the unidentified object.

This mysterious object was never mentioned in the final autopsy report, which otherwise accounted for more than thirty-five metal particles from the bullet still left in Kennedy's head, many of which were the size of a grain of sand. Since the autopsy doctors did not publicly comment on this object and since the brain and slides that might show what it is are unavailable, Dr. Wecht only can guess that it could be one of several things—a hemorrhage caused by the gunshot wounds, or a piece of metal such as a bullet or bullet fragment, or a brain tumor, or some kind of vascular malformation.

Dr. Wecht does not believe that it is a hemorrhage caused by the gunshot wounds, for he says that if that were true, the doctors would have recorded it in the autopsy report. Moreover, he is convinced that because of its size, the three doctors could not have missed it. Its omission in the report therefore had to be deliberate.

If it is a bullet or the fragment of a bullet, it raises other questions, for there should not be another bullet or large fragment from a bullet still in Kennedy's head if only one gunman shot Kennedy twice.

If it is the third possibility, a brain tumor or some kind of vascular malformation, it raises still further questions. Did it affect the president in any way, or would it have ultimately affected him—and therefore perhaps the country—had he lived? Certainly the public should be curious about this mysterious object, but we may never know what it is, unless the brain or the slides of the brain are produced.

The autopsy photographs disclose another odd thing, a loose flap of skin on the *left* side and at the back of Kennedy's head. Amazingly enough, this too was not mentioned in the autopsy report. But tucked away in the twenty-seven volumes of the Warren Commission report is a short statement by a Dr. Marion Jenkins, who saw what appeared to be this same wound when Kennedy was brought into the Dallas hospital. Dr. Jenkins testified that it was bleeding at the time, which is significant because it means the wound was pre-mortem and probably had something to do with the shooting, as opposed to careless handling or transportation of Kennedy after his death. Based on Dr. Wecht's experience with more than 1,500 bullet wound cases, he believes the wound is too small to have been caused by a complete bullet but was caused, more likely, by a fragment of a shell.

If Kennedy was shot once in the back with the bullet traveling through to his throat, and again from the back and into the right side of his head, as the autopsy report and Warren Commission stated, then any destruction on the left side of the head would certainly appear suspicious. In fact, the wound should have been investigated at the time of the autopsy. Incredibly enough, however, the three doctors never made a thorough search of Kennedy's head to see whether more than one bullet struck him. It is usually standard in such cases to go through the hair carefully or shave off portions if necessary to see if—as occasionally happens—a bullet wound is hidden by the hair and is missed because it does not bleed. No such examination was made. But the damage to the left side of the head and Kennedy's leftward movement on the Zapruder film, which suggests he was struck from the right, seem inconsistent. If the missing brain were ever found, it might provide the missing link so that an accurate reconstruction of the assassination could be made.

Dr. Wecht's findings, statements, and accusations did not please a number of people, especially as he made headlines with them. Still, he remains an outspoken critic of the Warren Commission report, and even before he examined the evidence in the National Archives, he had written articles voicing his doubts about the official version of the assassination. As a result, he was not exactly welcomed with open arms when he asked for permission as a qualified medical expert to go to the National Archives. In August 1971 he wrote a letter to Burke Marshall, the Kennedy family lawyer (and the man who decides which doctors get to see the materials), requesting permission to view the evidence. Marshall replied that he would have to ask the National Archives, and when he did, they wrote him back and said he had to write to Marshall! Marshall pretty much ignored Wecht's letters for a year until Fred Graham of *The New York Times* expressed interest in doing a story on the runaround Wecht was being given. At that point, the material was made available to Wecht.

Before Dr. Wecht examined the evidence, the Ramsey Clark panel of three medical detectives and a radiologist (Dr. William Carnes, Dr. Russell Fisher, Dr. R. H. Morgan, Dr. Alan Moritz) also analyzed the assassination materials. Later, permission to view the evidence was granted to a urologist who claims to be a ballistics expert on the Kennedy assassination. (The choice of this man annoyed a number of medical detectives, including one who asked to remain nameless who said: "The only time a urologist should have been allowed to analyze this stuff would be if Oswald had urinated on Kennedy from the sixth floor of the Texas School Book Depository.") The decision to let a urologist come to conclusions in the area of forensic pathology may have been posited on the fact that he had written several articles supporting the Warren Commission conclusion before seeing the evidence.

It is certainly unfortunate that the doctors who performed the original autopsy made so many errors and left out so many crucial things in their report that others find their conclusions less than substantial. This may be related to the special fields of these doctors. While the first two members of the team were pathologists, they were hospital, not forensic, pathologists. Medical detection was not their area of expertise. The distinction between hospital and forensic pathology is not artificial. Forensic pathology (i.e., medical detection) is recognized by the American Board of Pathology as a sub-specialty, and special examinations are required in this area. The fields differ because while hospital pathologists do autopsies, they usually deal with natural rather than violent deaths. They are generally called upon to confirm or refute diagnoses made by doctors before their patients' deaths and they usually do not concern themselves with the how-was-it-done and other collateral information that will be used in a court of law. Thus it is not surprising that the chief hospital pathologist in the JFK assassination, Dr. James J. Humes, had had previous experience with only one bullet wound case, although what was surprising was that he was not only asked to make the autopsy but to head the team.

Only one of the three men, Dr. Pierre Finck, was a forensic pathologist, but his experience seems to have been limited to reviewing other people's cases rather than working on bullet wound cases himself. Furthermore, he was handicapped by arriving after the autopsy had already started (he was called only after the other two began work and realized they needed a forensic pathologist) and his authority may well have been limited, being an army doctor working with two navy doctors in a naval hospital.

Still, although the three doctors made a number of mistakes (such as probing a bullet wound with their fingers) and did a lot of unorthodox things (such as lining up wounds in relation to obscure parts of the body, the positions of which vary among individuals) they may have done a better job than believed. It is possible that they may not have been permitted to release all of their findings, that their report may have been changed later, and that they were under some control during the autopsy. Actually, they definitely were under some control, for at the Clay Shaw trial in New Orleans, when District Attorney Jim Garrison asked Dr. Finck why the doctors had not performed the standard task of dissecting the wound in Kennedy's back during the autopsy in order to determine the path of the bullet, Finck replied, "We were told not to." Not dissecting that wound was a great mistake, for it would have shown whether the bullet that supposedly entered from the back really traversed Kennedy's body and came out in the front of the neck—or perhaps vice versa—or whether the shot in Kennedy's back and the one in his throat were the result of two different bullets, one from the front and one from the back.

After the report was completed, sections were deleted. Admiral George Burkley, Kennedy's personal physician, received the report immediately after its completion and he has admitted that he only revealed those portions that he considered "necessary." Two months after he released these portions, the Secret Service received the report, and two months after them, the FBI. So the only autopsy report that ever told the entire story was the first one. But the American public may never learn what that said. Perhaps the oddest, most unconventional aspect of the entire autopsy was that the first autopsy report that was written—the one that said where the bullets entered and exited, where the wounds were located, how many bullets there were, their paths, and whether any still remain in Kennedy—was burned by Dr. Humes right after he wrote it.

It is possible that the reason that portions of the autopsy report and Kennedy's brain are missing has nothing to do with withholding evidence that would "prove a conspiracy." It was a source of speculation before Kennedy's death that he suffered from Addison's disease, a rare ailment caused by chronic insufficiency of hormone production in the adrenal glands. These rumors were given credence in 1967 when it came out that an article in a 1955 *Archives of Surgery Journal* described a man of Kennedy's age who suffered from Addison's disease and who underwent identical back surgery at the exact same time and in the same hospital as Kennedy. To add to the coincidence, this man had had a second operation four months later, as did Kennedy, and again in the same hospital for the same back condition.

Besides the puffiness in Kennedy's face, which was pronounced at his death and which some people speculate could have resulted from cortisone taken to curb the ailment; and in addition to Kennedy's deep suntan, which some say was the discoloration caused by this disease (others say he kept himself suntanned to hide the discoloration), the autopsy report implied that Kennedy had some kind of adrenal problems—mostly by what it *did not* say.

Although it is standard in an autopsy report to discuss the condition of every gland in the body in order to rule out all the possible what-done-its, Kennedy's report did not mention his adrenal glands. Not that the doctors did not notice them, for Dr. J. Thornton Boswell admitted five years later that they had identified and examined the adrenal glands at the autopsy.

"That proves they were diseased," says Dr. Wecht, "because if they were healthy, they would have been glad to say so and end the rumors."

If Kennedy had Addison's disease, and an attempt was made to hide it, it could explain why certain things were missing from the Archives or not discussed in the autopsy report: for example, the large object on the right side of Kennedy's brain could have been a benign or malignant tumor that caused his adrenal problems.

The real answer is to be found in the brain and all the other medical evidence.

But these are speculations which may never be satisfied, because the parts of the body that could prove or disprove them—the brain—is missing, together with vital portions of the autopsy report. Withholding or altering information has fostered exactly what the public and the government would have preferred ended: rumors, theories, and insinuations of conspiracy.

17

Dr. John Edland: Attica Revisited

There is not time to present an in-depth study of the riot that took place at Attica prison in September of 1971. Some background is necessary, however, in order to understand the significant role played by a young medical detective named Dr. John Edland. Like most medical detectives, he witnessed the end product of today's violent society and reported his findings in an unbiased manner to the public. In so doing, he may have changed the course of American history.

The troubles at Attica Correctional Facility near Buffalo, New York, began on September 9, 1971. They may have started technically when an officer was struck in the head by a soup can in retaliation for sending two prisoners to solitary. Or they may have started when another officer went to speak to the prisoners involved and was knocked to the floor.

But the roots of the riot were planted long before that. Like most prisons in America today, "correctional facility" is a misnomer. The fifty-three-acre maximum-security prison is really just another place to lock away and forget those whom society has failed to help earlier.

Imprisoned at Attica, isolated by a thirty-foot-high wall capped with fourteen gun-towers, are some of the most embittered and violent convicts in the country, most of whom are treated like animals. Before the uprising, the prisoners spent fourteen to sixteen hours a day in cells six feet by nine feet, and when they were let out to work, their jobs were often degrading and demeaning. Since there were too many prisoners for the available jobs, for example, they would have to sweep an already clean floor over and over. They were paid from thirty cents to one dollar a day, an improvement over the 1970 rate of six to twenty-nine cents a day, but little consolation to those who worked in the "slave shop," the metal shop, where temperatures reached almost 90 degrees. These men watched the materials they made for thirty-five cents a day bring in profits of $150,000 a year for the prison system.

Although eight million dollars was spent in 1971 for the upkeep of Attica and the inmates, less than 5 percent went to their wages; only 8.5 percent was allocated for food, medical supplies, and the clothing that was hot in summer and cold in winter. Only sixty-three cents a day was budgeted for each inmate's food, and not surprisingly, it failed to meet minimum dietary standards set forth by the federal government.

The men were allowed one roll of toilet paper and one bar of soap a month; replacements had to be bought—along with toothbrushes, toothpaste, razors, blades, and other essentials—from their "income," which averaged seven to seven and a half dollars a month. Moreover, they could buy it only at the commissary, where prices were comparable to those outside. (Fortunately for the men, they were able to make some of the products they needed on their own and hustle them among themselves. Pornography was hand-drawn and sold. Moonshine was made from fermented potatoes, rice, juices, and yeast usually stolen from the bakery. Drugs were slipped out of the hospital by hiding them under the prisoners' tongues. And shivs were made by many of the prisoners who wanted to protect themselves from the ubiquitous prison homosexuals.)

The men complained that not only were they frequently "corrected" with solitary confinement, but were punished additionally by beatings on the way. Once in solitary, they said they were given one bucket for food and another for use as a toilet; when the buckets were emptied and returned, they never knew which was which.

The list of indignities at Attica, as at nearly all prisons, are endless, but one of Attica's biggest problems cannot be overlooked: of more than 2,200 inmates, only 37 percent were white; of 383 guards, not one was black. Moreover, the better jobs went to the whites. Segregation was rampant. There were white and black sports teams, different barbers for blacks and whites. As one black prisoner who had been stationed in Mississippi and Alabama in the army commented: "I have never seen so much discrimination [as in Attica]."

However the problems started, wherever they started, by nine-fifteen A.M. on September 9, the prison alarm was sounded and soon almost half of the prisoners were embroiled in a full-scale riot. Most of those outside the prison, especially those who lived in the tiny town of Attica, failed to realize the seriousness of the situation and viewed it as more of a carnival than a riot. Some of the residents even stood outside to watch the "fun," and one entrepreneur set up a hamburger stand for the onlookers.

But the prisoners weren't playing around. Twelve hundred of them seized control of Cell Block D plus portions of another, and fashioned weapons in the machine shop from baseball bats, hammers, clubs, pipes and spears made from scissor blades (after the riot 1,400 weapons were found in the prison). Portions of the prison were wrecked, some for purposes of defense, others perhaps in an inarticulate plea for help. The hoses of the prison firefighting equipment were shredded; the windows were broken; the wire fence was electrified; and several buildings, including the church and school, were burned down, although ironically later demands included better schooling and more religious freedom. Most important, 43 guards were grabbed and held as hostage.

Some of these guards were immediately injured, including 28-year-old William Quinn, who was allegedly tossed out of a window by the prisoners. Although the prisoners released him and some other injured guards to the medical authorities, the remaining guards were not so lucky. They were blindfolded, stripped, and garbed in inmate's clothes. With these hostages, the prisoners were in a good position to demand improvement of their deplorable condition.

The prisoners insisted on things which they should have been granted years before, such as an increase in pay. (Why cannot prisoners earn minimum wages and then give a portion to their victims as restitution?) They asked for permission to hold political meetings, religious freedom, increased educational facilities, an end to mail censorship, and an improved diet containing more fresh fruit and less pork, the latter in deference to the religious beliefs of the incarcerated Black Muslims. Some wanted immediate transportation to nonimperialistic countries, and they all asked a promise of amnesty in addition to the ouster of Vincent Mancusi, the prison superintendent, who on the first day of the uprising asked: "Why are they destroying their home?"

Russell Oswald, the New York commissioner of correctional services, agreed to twenty-eight of the thirty demands, but the prisoners did not believe his promise that there would be no retaliation for the riot. And during the negotiations, something happened that made them far less concerned with minor concessions, and even more worried about possible retaliation. William Quinn, the prison guard who had been pushed out of the window, died from his injuries. And what good was an end to mail censorship or less pork if the prisoners later found themselves in death row?

As their truculence increased, things became even more dangerous. Each hostage was assigned to a prison "executioner," who stood by ready to kill him. But the prisoners seemed to realize the danger of their situation, and asked Governor Rockefeller to come in. The hostages were even more anxious for him to intercede in the riot, for as one of them said, "Unless Rockefeller comes, I am a dead man." The Governor refused to come; the next day, that guard's prophesy came true.

Early on the morning of September 14, approximately 500 police, state troopers, sheriffs, and deputies stood outside the prison. Ready. Meanwhile, helicopters carrying tear gas circled above; and all available ambulances and National Guardsmen in the area were waiting nearby. At seven-forty A.M., Oswald again urged the prisoners in a written memorandum to release their captives. Only one prisoner spoke out in favor of accepting (although later many said they had wanted to) and the response of the others was to have the executioners march the eight blindfolded and bound hostages out with knives positioned at their throats.

Oswald decided to act. At nine-forty-four came the order to attack; although the instructions allegedly were to "shoot only to prevent death or injury to one of our own or to the hostages." That was not what happened. Rifles burst from the top of the turreted prison walls. Tear gas was dropped by the helicopters. And several hundred state police with gas masks, high-powered rifles, sidearms, and 12-gauge shotguns charged in. Although the full, one-sided battle (only one trooper was injured) took less than fifteen minutes, it was, as the McKay Commission reported, the bloodiest one-day encounter between Americans since the Civil War. During the attack, the police confused hostages and inmates because the guards were wearing prisoner's uniforms. The "liberators' " vision also was hindered on that dark morning by gas masks (these inhibited verbal communication as well) and by the rain, as well as the tear gas that was falling from the sky. Furthermore, the state police had been forbidden to engage in hand-to-hand combat for fear that the prisoners would seize their guns. They kept shooting, therefore, without looking at or getting close to their prey. And so—no one knew how—some of the hostages were killed.

When it was over, thirty-nine were dead: ten hostages and twenty-nine inmates; and three hostages and eighty-five inmates were wounded. Others were injured by vicious and deliberate beatings after the "battle"—despite the promise of no physical retaliation. (Oswald testified later that he heard that the law officers were "merely prodding them with their batons on the buttocks [and not] striking them. . . . It was much like a fraternity hazing.")

Later, the death toll rose to forty-three and the exact number of injured probably never will be known. The state immediately placed the blame for the guards' death on the prisoners, and Deputy Commissioner Walter Dunbar announced that they had slit the hostages' throats, that one of the guards had been emasculated and his testicles stuffed in his mouth: statements that all have been criticized sharply. The rumors may have stemmed from a severe gunshot wound in the groin suffered by one of the hostages, though Dunbar went so far as to say that the "castration" had been filmed from a helicopter.

On September 14, everyone knew that something terrible had happened at Attica, but until Dr. John Edland, the medical detective, stepped in, no one realized just how bad things really were. He established beyond question that the guards had been killed by the very people who had been sent in to save them.

Dr. John Frederic Edland, the chief medical examiner of Monroe County, observed the Attica riots from the beginning. Today he does not like to talk about what happened during those tense days. Furthermore, he resents the public's obsessive interest in just one of his cases, when he has handled many others well. He cringes when people accidentally introduce him as "Dr. Attica," or say that he lives in "Attica, New York." ("Rochester, Rochester," he hisses.)

When Edland was thrust into the limelight after Attica, it was not totally alien to him: he had achieved renown back in his high school days as a football player. Indeed, football was indirectly responsible for his choice of a career; when a leg injury from football prevented him from going out for the college team, he turned to study, and unable to decide between law or medicine as a career, he chose both by becoming a medical examiner. He was not only a high-scoring football player; he also scored well with girls. He had no problem in getting five of them to say yes to his offers of marriage—not all at the same time, of course. Fortunately for him, he only followed through on one of them, and married a pretty blonde who, like her husband, winces at being introduced as "Mrs. Attica."

Edland realized from the beginning that the uprising at Attica would mean work for him. He described the incident as follows:

"I became more and more concerned as the week went on. It became increasingly obvious that there was a national problem here, similar to what happened at Kent State. I knew that if anything serious occurred I would immediately be called in, and I lived in dread that week. I'm a very private person, although I'll admit I've chosen a flamboyant profession. The last thing I wanted was to suddenly find myself in the limelight.

"I guess my feelings about that were based partly on personal reasons, but there were business ones, too. Things have gone well for me and I've built up a good reputation among my colleagues. [Dr. Edland is one of the youngest of the medical detectives. Three years before Attica, at the age of thirty-three, he became the chief medical examiner of Monroe County, an area with a population of 750,000 people. He performs six hundred autopsies each year. While most medical examiners at thirty-three are still working for others, Edland had thirty-two staff people working under him.] I've worked hard for it, but I knew that all I've accomplished could be destroyed in the time that it takes to do an autopsy if I made a mistake with the press and the world looking on. Look what people said about the pathologist who did the Kennedy autopsy. Or the handwriting expert on the Hughes-Irving case."

Edland speaks in a slow, deliberate fashion; his answers to questions are drawn out of him.

"All medical examiners and forensic experts in general have to live with the same fear now: that an entire career, with all the years of study it required, can be ruined in a minute if someone rightly criticizes our findings on an important case."

"Therefore, most of us dread the death of a national figure in our jurisdiction because the most incredible pressure then ensues with the press and the public. Besides which, there's also the simply physical and mental anguish of an important autopsy. It has to be handled with kid gloves. The hardest are the homicidal cases, and when you've got a killing by gun, it's murder for us as well as the victim. First of all, you have to find the bullet, or more often the bullets, as well as all the pieces that may have broken off in the body. Then you've got to establish where the entrance and exit wound is for each bullet, chart the course of the bullet through the body, and also do the same for any pieces of the bullet that may have broken off and remain lodged in the body. After that, you've got to look for additional wounds, and then perform all the regular tasks of an autopsy. Multiply that by many people with several bullets in them and it's torture. Although I realized then that a few people might get shot at Attica, little did I realize just how many homicides would be involved—and one of the victims had twelve bullets in him.

"Naturally, when you've got only a small number of

victims your job is much easier. Kennedy's death was an extremely difficult autopsy to do, but it was still an autopsy of just one person. The Tate autopsy must have been a gruesome and difficult job for Noguchi, but it was four bodies to work on. I had the uncomfortable feeling all along that the Attica toll might even be higher than that, but I never imagined that it would eventually reach forty-three.

"But I began to see the handwriting on the wall when they called to tell me that William Quinn had died. He was the guard who had been pushed down the stairs. [It was reported, as noted earlier, that the inmates had tossed him out of the window, but many questioned whether this was possible, since there were bars on the windows.] He lingered a couple of days before dying, and the cause of death was finally attributed to head injuries, although there was some dispute about that. When I heard he was dead, I suspected my troubles were starting.

"I was sure of it the next day when it was announced that the police had been called in to quell the riot. While most people who heard that news probably put down their newspapers, or turned off their TV sets and went on with whatever they had been doing, I sat and waited. I knew it was just a matter of time then before the phone would start ringing for me. There were only two forensic pathologists in that whole section of New York and I was one of them. It was inevitable. Later I found out that they did call two physicians in that area, but those doctors said it would take weeks to autopsy so many victims. So the two doctors only took five cases each, and I was stuck with the rest. It was about ten in the morning when I started waiting for the call and I waited all day. It was one of those deathly quiet days when probably not even a salesman called.

"But at six P.M. the telephone rang. It was the captain of the state police asking me if I was willing to take all the cases I could possibly handle since there had been a mass disaster. I agreed, but only under one condition: I wanted to autopsy *all* of the guards. There were already some questions brewing as to how they had died, and whether their throats had really been slashed by the prisoners who were holding them as hostages. I knew that only if I examined all the guards would I be able to come to a conclusion about what had really happened to them. I certainly didn't think that they had died of bad air, but I had also read some horrifying reports that they had been mutilated and their genitals stuffed in their mouths. That sort of thing. I knew that if the cases were spread out, and one doctor did one guard, and another doctor took others, it might be years before the truth would ever come out. In retrospect, keeping the guards together was one of the best decisions I've ever made.

"At twelve-ten in the morning they started to bring in twenty-seven bodies, eighteen hostages and nine inmates. They brought them into the garage in two large trucks, and the medical photographer who was supposed to photograph them all took one look at the carnage and practically went into shock. 'It's like finding twenty-seven dead people in your garage,' he said. Although the guards and the prisoners were dressed the same way, I could tell the difference because the guards had tags with their names on them, and all had their hands tied behind their backs. Some had their feet bound as well. But the prisoners were simply toe-tagged P-1 through P-18 [Prisoner 1, etc.].

"The whole atmosphere was very emotional, which made it extremely hard to work. A convoy of state police had been sent to guard the office. I don't know why or what anyone was afraid might happen. I've heard of lots of places being stormed but never a morgue. Anyway, I had agreed to do twenty-seven of the bodies, and since there were only two slabs and twenty stretchers, we set up an assembly line, or as one reporter wrote later, a 'dis-assembly line.'

"Each person was brought in, weighed, measured, superficially examined, and fingerprinted. Usually I wait to do fingerprinting until later, but in this case I wanted to make sure that the guards really were who they were supposed to be.

"Before I started working on them I also had to figure out which of the bodies needed to be X-rayed to look for broken bones or concealed weapons. Once I started autopsying, Richard Abbott, my deputy, and I were bouncing back and forth trying to split cases. Someone else was in another room developing the photographs. People were shouting all around. You couldn't take a break or relax for a minute.

"On top of it, the smell was terrible, not from death, but from the CS gas [O-Chlorobenzalononitrile] which they had dropped from the helicopters. Although the bodies had been washed before they got to me, there was just no getting rid of it. It made my eyes tear, my skin burn, and I felt like I was having an asthmatic attack. Some of the others had to leave because of it, and as a result we worked with a reduced staff. I had called in all off-duty people, but there still weren't enough. I felt as if I was working almost alone on twenty-seven bodies, which is more than I ever want to see in one day. This field has always been my whole life to me, and that day was definitely the worst day of my life. There were eighty-seven hours of solid work, although a regular simple autopsy usually takes about one hour."

Dr. Edland described his usual procedure:

"The first thing I do when I make an autopsy is to check the body for external deformities, wounds, lividity, etc. I like to examine the body first with clothes on because the clothes often tell you something. Rings, the type of apparel worn, whether it's torn, what's in the pockets. That's all important. I usually don't make fingerprints until after the autopsy is completed, because first I do tests for nitrate on the hands [to see if the dead man recently shot a gun], check for injection marks to see if he was an addict, look for subtle tattoos such as the one homosexuals wear between their thumb and index finger, and things like that. If they've been strangled and the ligature is still on them, I don't untie it but cut it off at the sides so that later I can study how it was tied.

"Once they're undressed I look for wounds, scars, and bruises. With these people, I also tested each wound for gunpowder by placing some specially-treated tape into the wound. I didn't find any gunpowder—showing that none of the people had been shot at close range.

"The next step is the actual autopsy. I make the usual Y-shaped incision, which is popular in America and was started by the Germans in order to prevent destroying the breasts. It starts at the shoulders, goes under the breasts, and then straight down to the pubis. Then I lift the skin back, pull away the muscles and fat, remove the breast plate, and open up the abdominal and chest cavity so that everything is exposed. Then I take out each organ individually and look for diseases, trauma, and physical abnormalities caused by external factors such as knives or bullets. I also take out any bullets I find and they're placed in plastic cups with the case number on it. During all this time, I'm describing what I find into a dictaphone with a microphone hung from the ceiling so my hands are free to work.

"At the end of the autopsy I make a provisional diagnosis, put everything back in, and sew the body up with a sailing needle, the type that's used for canvas. The tissues go to histology for microscopic sections; the blood, bile, urine, liver, kidney, and stomach contents go to toxicology. Some of the blood goes to serology for grouping and typing, and swabs from the anus, vagina, and sometimes the mouth are also sent to serology to check for semen. During the whole procedure photographs are being taken, and a provisional certificate is then signed."

For these autopsies, Dr. Edland decided to begin on the guards. The dead guards were the heroes, and inside the prison their colleagues were taking vengeance. On one occasion five or six correction officers used nightsticks to beat a prisoner lying naked on the floor. He was carried out on a stretcher, delirious, repeating, "I didn't do it, boss." The man had abrasions and lacerations on his elbows, buttocks, back, and scalp. But when asked about the incident, one of the officers involved said: "He was pushed to some extent because he wasn't responding normally . . . he simply went the wrong way and fell . . . and he hit his head either on the door or the door handle or something at the bottom of the stairs."

"I looked at the first guard," Edland continued, "and saw his neck all covered with blood and that he had a really bad head wound. Actually, his whole head was shattered. Based on the blood, the wounds, and the information I had received, I figured that he'd probably been bludgeoned to death by his executioner.

"Just as I was starting to work on him, the X-ray technician came running in to bring me the print he had just developed of the man. He didn't run because he realized the implications of that X-ray; he ran because we were working so fast. He hadn't even had time to look at the X-ray. We had made it just to look for broken bones and concealed weapons. We didn't expect anything else.

"I was the first to look at it and couldn't believe what I saw. In his head was a huge slug. I took in a breath and just kept staring at that X-ray. 'My God,' I realized. 'This guard wasn't stabbed to death, as they said: he was obviously shot to death.' Of course the implications were also immediately obvious: since none of the inmates had guns, the guard could only have been killed by the police. My suspicion about what he had died from was confirmed when I washed away the blood which had dripped from his head wound, and there were no neck wounds on the guard whatsoever.

"I thought maybe that was just a freak. He probably accidentally got in the way of the police. And then I began to work on the next guard. And the next one after that. The story was the same. *Every one* had been shot to death. It was overkill. I was unhappy enough over what I saw, but I was also worried about what I was going to say about it. I kept thinking that a lot of people were going to be very depressed over what I had found. After all, the state police were supposed to shoot the executioners, and save the guards—not the other way around.

"Meanwhile, besides examining the bullets and wounds, there was additional work to be done. Many people there were running around spreading stories like 'the niggers were screwing them in the ass.' I knew the rumors were ridiculous. Who has time during an assault to bother sodomizing? But the rumors had to be checked. My suspicion was correct. I never found any semen.

"There was also another job that had to be done. Although most of the work I did on each person was the same, there were two exceptions. Two of the prisoners the police were especially interested in, because one had been found in a hole and another in a cell block. It appeared that they had been executed earlier and died before the assault on the prison. To determine if this was true, I checked their body temperatures. The attack had occurred in the morning and all the other people had body temperatures of between eighty-four and eighty-six degrees. But I found that these two were at seventy-seven degrees, which confirmed that they were killed before the others.

"I took a break sometime during that night but I couldn't sleep. I just lay there and looked at the ceiling. At around nine in the morning, I went back to work. I kept waiting for someone else to announce the truth to the forty or so state policemen around, but no one said anything. Not one word. I don't think any of them there actually realized the implications of those bullets because they continued to discuss the slashing of the guards' throats.

"But the press began to realize that something was happening. One of our local reporters learned what I had found and my work was constantly being interrupted. People kept coming in to tell me that every radio and TV station in the country was on the phone and they wanted to know when they could send their crews up. I couldn't take the time out to stop and talk to each of them so I set up a press conference at three P.M. Actually, I *did* talk to one of them separately from the others. About an hour before my press conference, someone came running in to tell me that there was a call from Rockefeller's press information office in Albany. A man came on the phone with a voice like John Foster Dulles and identified himself as Governor Rockefeller's personal secretary. He asked me what the entire story was, and of course I told him. Then he said, 'Doctor, the governor appreciates your candor,' and hung up. I never did find out who the jerk was, but he turned out not to be anyone from Rockefeller's office. He was probably a reporter trying to jump the story by an hour.

"I had figured that just the local Rochester media and a couple of bigger stations might come this way for the conference so I put on a nondescript outfit and my good-luck coat, which had cost me twenty-eight dollars, and prepared to walk out. I glanced out first, and discovered that it was so packed that there wasn't enough room for me. It looked like hundreds of people and thousands of microphones out there. Like a press conference for Nixon. I hadn't even planned on what I was going to say, so it ended up as a completely unrehearsed press conference. I was quite embarrassed though before I walked out, because a public relations information officer marched up and dramatically announced to the press, 'Ladies and gentlemen—the medical examiner of Monroe County.' The guy had obviously seen too many presidential press conferences.

"And then I walked out and faced a multitude of staring people. Somehow, I felt like I was back at the old football games again. Everyone was watching and waiting to see what I would do next. Someone put a piece of paper on the floor and told me to stand on that. I did and looked out and saw that the New York press corps had pushed our little local guys all the way to the back. They still complain about it to this day.

"And then I made a statement. I explained that the autopsies showed that all the hostages had been killed by guns. That caused an immediate stir since it was known that only the police, not the prisoners, had guns. I explained that the earlier announcement that they had died by knives and beatings was wrong, although some did bear marks of beatings. But none of these had been severe enough to kill them. They died from bullets, and some had been shot only once, but others five, ten, and even twelve times. Some were even shot in the back. One guard had a single cut in the back of his neck, but he, like the rest, died from gunshot wounds. Two of the *prisoners*, on the other hand, had died of slashed throats and multiple stab wounds. No one had been castrated.

"When it was over, there was quite a bit of excitement, but it was nothing compared to the clamor that it caused later. To see little me headlined on page one: 'Doc says Guards Shot.' Or to see my picture under the lead in *The New York Times*! It was just incredible. My mother's still impressed.

"After the press conference, I went back to the autopsies and at six that night the police came running in shouting, 'Dr. Edland, Dr. Edland. You're on CBS.' I thought it was a joke and I came in rather reluctantly to watch myself. But there I was. I felt very self-conscious, you know, like you're watching someone else. Later I went home and decided to forget about the whole thing. I still had many more prisoners to autopsy but I figured the clamor over my announcement was over and I was glad.

"But about a half hour after I returned to my house, the state policeman in charge of the morgue detail called and said Dr. Henry Siegel from Westchester County had been called in to come up and review my findings. Then later I got another call that Mike Baden from the New York office had also been called and was coming in. Later, they had The Chief [Helpern] review my autopsy findings. The higher-ups in Albany just didn't want to believe what I had found, so they were sending in other medical examiners to confirm it, although I guess they were really hoping they'd deny it."

The commissioners also tried to prove that the "foreign projectiles" that Edland wrote about in his report, referring to bullets, were in fact bombs constructed by the prisoners. Five National Guard teams with mine detectors were sent in to search for bombs and buried weapons, while Edland, who had voted for Goldwater in 1964, was categorized as a "clown" and a "radical left-winger."

"Dr. Siegel spent that first night checking my findings and Baden came in the next morning. It was a little difficult for them to do the job, though, because after I'd completed each autopsy, the bodies had been sent to local funeral homes. So the bodies of the guards were scattered all over the area. Actually, had it been my jurisdiction I would have *invited* them to come in. But I was a little surprised that all of these people were just being sent in without my being asked about it. But I guess I was kind of glad, too. After all, they didn't find anything I hadn't.

"Later some of the guards' burials were held up while people were still trying to find the slashed throats. Even today, there are people who are *still* trying to find something different. One of the guards had a scratch on his throat. Now they're trying to say that that scratch killed him. Not the two bullets in his head. It's ridiculous. Many people in the town of Attica still refuse to believe that the guards were killed by gunshots, and that none were castrated. In fact, right after Attica, a rumor circulated through the town that some *living* guards as well as the dead ones had been castrated by the prisoners.

"A few days after the completion of my autopsies, some undertaker signed an affidavit saying that there had been no gunshot wounds on one of the guards whose death I had attributed to shooting. I had just moved and the TV crews set up cameras and floodlights in front of my former home to photograph the empty place as if I had skipped town. Mike Baden was still up here and he went over to examine the guard who had supposedly died of a slashed throat. The guard was lying on his back so that you couldn't see the bullet hole. Baden turned him over and there was the wound, right in the back. The undertaker was out bowling so he called him back. When he arrived, Baden pointed to the hole and asked him, 'What's that?' 'A bullet hole,' he admitted. And that was the end of that.

"But I guess this all shows how things have changed in our job. I am my own man. I call the shots as I see them and I'm used to not finding what people tell me I will find. In releasing the information, I felt that I might be saving lives. But there are many who feel that information damaging to the government should be kept secret. The medical examiner was traditionally on the side of the government and law enforcement. But it's just not true anymore. We are now an independent medico-legal organization. We're not interested in the prosecution or defense of any case. We just report what we find, and the only side we're on now is the side of truth."

Ombudsmen of Death

Although most of this book has concentrated on individual cases usually involving violence, this is only a small segment of what the medical detectives do. In addition to investigating murder, they must look into all suspicious, unexplained, and even some natural deaths.

As a result, the medical detectives' findings affect not only criminology cases but the general population as well. There are hundreds of examples of lives saved because the medical detectives figured out why only a few died. To cite just a few cases: when penicillin was first introduced, it was hailed as a panacea and prescribed as casually and indiscriminately as aspirin. It was a medical detective in Manhattan, Dr. Abraham Rosenthal, who discovered that the people he was autopsying could not have died from the disease for which the penicillin had been prescribed. For example, one girl casually was given penicillin for a "sprained toe." The only possible what-done-it was the penicillin. As a result, doctors exercised more caution in prescribing this drug.

It was a medical detective, Dr. Elliot Gross, chief

medical examiner of Connecticut, who autopsied the victims of an early Boeing 727 plane crash, and concluded that the cause of death was not injuries from the accident, but burns from the fire in which they were trapped. As a result of his report, the 727 was redesigned to reduce the chances of people being trapped in an airplane fire.

It was a medical detective, Dr. Alexander Wiener, director of serological and bacteriological laboratories in the Office of the Chief Medical Examiner of Manhattan, who was co-discoverer of the Rh-factor in blood, and who became aware that babies from Rh-negative mothers often died at birth. His findings led to precautionary methods prior to delivery which have saved the lives of thousands of infants.

Most of the work of the medical detectives is not nearly this dramatic, as Dr. Werner Spitz, the medical examiner of Wayne County, Michigan, points out. Forensic medicine does not involve heroic heart and kidney transplants; it is a slow but steady work. In fact most of the "new developments" in forensic medicine are borrowed and applied from medicine. On the other hand, the results return in the form of assistance to medical research, doctors, and patients, for uncovering the cause of death often can aid in the prescription and treatment of other patients. Yet, in the United States, little such research is done. Only 30 percent of all patients who die in hospitals are autopsied, as opposed to 80 percent in England and 100 percent in Russia.

Obviously, if there were more medical detectives to perform autopsies, society would be the better. But the profession is not growing as fast as it should, and many medical detectives complain that in general it is not attracting the competent American medical students.

There are fewer than 100 qualified, full-time forensic pathologists in the United States at the present time and only about 10 or 15 new ones each year. Yet this is not the only area where medico-legal experts are needed.

While forensic pathologists are necessary to examine the cause and manner of death, identify human remains, or study the relationship between trauma and injury to disease, forensic toxicologists are needed to study poison in relation to crime and occupational diseases, to do chemical tests to determine intoxication; forensic psychiatrists are needed to study the pattern of crimes and criminals, or to accrue evidence of insanity for a defense; forensic serologists are needed to work on blood for paternity suits, immigration requirements, identification of victims and assailants; forensic odontologists are needed to examine teeth and bite marks.

One reason that medical students (and Ph.D. candidates) shy away from forensic medicine is its low pay. Another is its incredibly hard work. They cannot just knock off and play golf on Wednesdays. As Dr. Sidney Weinberg, medical examiner of Suffolk County, says, "This is a twenty-four-hours-a-day, seven-days-a-week job. People just don't die by appointment." And when a medical detective gets a call in the middle of the night, he or she cannot suggest that the patient take two aspirins and call back in the morning. The rapid degeneration makes it imperative that the body be examined immediately. Dr. James Luke, chief medical examiner of Washington, D.C., says, "We usually have only one chance to find the truth. There's just no putting Humpty Dumpty back together again after that."

William T. Curran, professor of legal medicine at Harvard Medical School, lists four trends in America that necessitate an increase in medical detection. The first and most obvious problem is the rise in violent deaths in America today, and most medical detectives agree that crimes are getting more complicated and sophisticated, making them harder to solve. Second is the spread of drugs and drug abuse. Third is an increasing hostility on the part of the public toward law-enforcement officials, which often makes it distrust the official explanations of cause and method of death. And the last is the increase in assassination.

These are disturbing problems, and the medical detectives are facing them already. They are keenly aware that they are in a position to do something good about the evils they see each day. Several of the medical detectives have been instrumental in getting laws enacted which help to prevent certain kinds of deaths. Others, like Dr. John Edland, believe that the way to change things is to publicize them, as he did with his findings at Attica. As he says, "I like to think that in theory many deaths can be prevented, and the way to do this is by informing the public about them. If not for hammering away daily about the number of deaths from drugs, it would have taken a lot longer before people even realized that there was a problem. We must get these tragedies before the people, even though it may be misconstrued as publicity-seeking or self-aggrandizement. But if we keep our cases to ourselves, or 'museum collect,' as we call it, hoard our slides and findings and discuss them only with other medical examiners, we're not really helping anyone. This country's on a real death-denial kick and only if we're educated to the evils that exist will we all be able to survive."

In addition to legislative change and public education, Dr. Michael Baden advocates doing more work on the *causes* of the problem. "It's not enough to dissect bodies and accumulate data," he says. "We must get involved in solving the problems that cause these deaths. A majority of deaths in young people in America today are from unnatural causes, such as drug addiction, suicide, car accidents, murder, child beatings, or abortions. All of these are potentially preventable, at least more so than natural diseases. But to prevent them, we should consider the parent as well as the beaten child, the automobile along with the driver. It doesn't do any good to call attention to the deaths if society doesn't do anything about the factors responsible."

The work of the medical detectives is the first step. They find the cause of death (what-done-it) and the manner of death (how-was-it-done). The media focuses attention on the problems that the medical detectives have uncovered. And then the public must care enough to do something about it. But the beginning is right there at the end: death. The medical detectives act as the ombudsmen of death, the people who speak for the deceased in a world where more and more people are violently dying, and the living are constantly crying out for help.

Suggested Readings

Browne, Douglas G., and Fuller, E. V. *The Scalpel of Scotland Yard; The Life of Sir Bernard Spilsbury.* New York: E. P. Dutton, 1952.

Bailey, F. Lee. *The Defense Never Rests.* New York: Stein and Day, 1971.

Carpozi, George, Jr. *Ordeal by Trial; The Alice Crimmins Case.* New York: Walker, 1972.

Camps, Francis E. *Legal Medicine.* Baltimore: Williams & Wilkins, 1968.

Gonzales, Thomas A.; Vance, Morgan; Helpern, Milton; and Umberger, Charles. *Legal Medicine, Pathology and Toxicology.* New York: Appleton-Century-Crofts, 1954.

Gradwohl, Rutherford, *Gradwohl's Legal Medicine.* Baltimore: Williams & Wilkins, 1968.

Gribble, Leonard. *Famous Feats of Detection and Deduction.* New York: Doubleday, Doran, 1934.

Gustafson, Gösta. *Forensic Odontology.* New York: American Elsevier, 1966.

Helfer, Ray E., and Kempe, Henry, eds. *The Battered Child.* Chicago: University of Chicago Press, 1968.

Houts, Marshall. *Where Death Delights; The Story of Milton Helpern and Forensic Medicine.* New York: Coward-McCann, 1967.

Jackson, Robert. *The Crime Doctors.* London: Frederick Muller, 1966.

Jones, Leland V. *Scientific Investigation and Physical Evidence.* Springfield, Ill.: C. C. Thomas, 1959.

Maine, C. E. *The World's Strangest Crimes.* New York: Hart, 1967.

Meagher, Sylvia. *Accessories after the Fact; the Warren Commission, the Authorities and the Report.* Indianapolis: Bobbs-Merrill, 1967.

Morland, Nigel, ed. *The Criminologist.* New York: Library Press, 1972.

————. *An Outline of Scientific Criminology.* London: Cassell, 1950.

Pollack, Jack Harrison. *Dr. Sam; An American Tragedy.* Chicago: Henry Regnery, 1972.

Polson, C. J. *The Scientific Aspects of Forensic Medicine.* Edinburgh: Oliver & Boyd, 1969.

Schatkin, Sidney. *Disputed Paternity Proceedings.* New York: Matthew Bender, 1967.

Smith, Sir Sydney. *Mostly Murder.* New York: David McKay, 1959.

Snyder, Lemoyne. *Homicide Investigation.* Springfield, Ill.: C. C. Thomas, 1950.

Thompson, Josiah. *Six Seconds in Dallas.* New York: Bernard Geis, 1968.

Thorwald, Jurgen. *Crime and Science.* New York: Harcourt Brace and World, 1967.

————. *The Century of the Detective.* New York: Harcourt Brace and World, 1965.

Tobin, Richard. *Golden Opinions.* New York: E. P. Dutton, 1948.

Watson, Eric B., ed. *The Trial of George Joseph Smith.* Edinburgh: W. Hodge, 1923.